Chicken Soup for the Soul®

Shaping the New You

Chicken Soup for the Soul: Shaping the New You
101 Encouraging Stories about Dieting and Fitness... and Finding What Works for You
Jack Canfield, Mark Victor Hansen, Amy Newmark. Foreword by Richard Simmons.

Published by Chicken Soup for the Soul Publishing, LLC   www.chickensoup.com
Copyright © 2010 by Chicken Soup for the Soul Publishing, LLC. All Rights Reserved.
No part of this publication may be reproduced, stored in a retrieval system or transmitted in any form or by any means, electronic, mechanical, photocopying, recording or otherwise, without the written permission of the publisher.

CSS, Chicken Soup for the Soul, and its Logo and Marks are trademarks of
Chicken Soup for the Soul Publishing LLC.

The publisher gratefully acknowledges the many publishers and individuals who
granted Chicken Soup for the Soul permission to reprint the cited material.

*Front cover photograph courtesy of iStockphoto.com/PhotoInc (© PhotoInc). Back cover photo
courtesy of Richard Simmons. Interior photo courtesy of iStockphoto.com/Erdosainview (© Julián
Rovagnati)*

Cover and Interior Design & Layout by Pneuma Books, LLC
For more info on Pneuma Books, visit www.pneumabooks.com

Distributed to the booktrade by Simon & Schuster. SAN: 200-2442

Publisher's Cataloging-in-Publication Data
(Prepared by The Donohue Group)

Chicken soup for the soul : shaping the new you : 101 encouraging stories about
  dieting and fitness-- and finding what works for you / [compiled by] Jack
  Canfield, Mark Victor Hansen, [and] Amy Newmark ; foreword by Richard Simmons.

    p. ; cm.

   Summary: A collection of 101 true personal stories from regular people about dieting
and fitness.
   ISBN: 978-1-935096-57-3

   1. Reducing diets--Literary collections. 2. Physical fitness--
Literary collections. 3. Health--Literary collections. 4. Reducing diets--
Anecdotes. 5. Physical fitness--Anecdotes. 6. Health--Anecdotes. I. Canfield, Jack,
1944- II. Hansen, Mark Victor. III. Newmark, Amy. IV. Simmons, Richard. V. Title:
Shaping the new you

PN6071.D52 C45 2010
810.8/02/03561   2010931657

PRINTED IN THE UNITED STATES OF AMERICA
on acid∞free paper
19 18 17 16 15 14 13 12 11 10   03 04 05 06 07 08 09 10

Chicken Soup for the Soul®

Shaping the New You

101 Encouraging Stories about Dieting and
Fitness... and Finding What Works for You

Jack Canfield,
Mark Victor Hansen,
Amy Newmark
Foreword by Richard Simmons

Chicken Soup for the Soul Publishing, LLC
Cos Cob, CT

Chicken Soup for the Soul

www.chickensoup.com

Contents

❶
~Getting Started~

❷
~Exercise Can Be Fun~

3

~To Err Is Human~

4

~Regaining Control~

5

~The Gym~

❻
~Liking Myself~

❼
~Having a Partner~

8

~Telling Myself the Truth~

9

~Foods that Made a Difference~

10

~Off the Beaten Path~

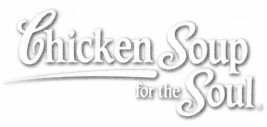

Foreword

My whole life is about inspiration, so when the folks from Chicken Soup for the Soul showed me the manuscript for this book about "Shaping the New You," I wanted to get involved. We all need some help when it comes to taking care of ourselves. We want to do it, we know how good it will feel to be in shape, but we need that push to do the hard work necessary to get there.

These 100 stories written by regular people about their efforts to control their weight and get fit really resonate with me. There is no better inspiration than hearing someone else's story. You will undoubtedly make a connection while reading this book—you'll find a little motivational trick that you know will work for you, or read a phrase that gets you out of your chair... and out of the kitchen!

No one has a bigger appetite than me! Food was my entire life growing up. I could be blindfolded and still find a po' boy place. I was raised in New Orleans, within walking distance of the best food in the world. I love food! But I have learned to love myself too. And that is how I dropped more than 100 pounds in my early twenties and kept it off for the four decades since.

My parents were in show business. Although they were larger than life, they had cute little bodies. I don't know if they had to work hard to look as good as they did. My mother was a professional singer and performer for much of my childhood. She was petite and always dressed elegantly—a real Auntie Mame type!

I was raised with music playing all the time in the house, and we lived around the corner from Preservation Hall. My parents danced in the living room. That is probably why exercising to music and dancing is so important to me.

My parents' philosophy was "Know no strangers." I use everything they taught me. No one remains a stranger to me. And it's funny how people will open up to me, on the most personal topics—their weight, their health, their life stories. I am like their priest or rabbi!

That's one of the things that I love about this book. The authors of these stories open up their lives to you and share their ups and downs (literally) and unselfishly pass on their wisdom. I am sure you will find useful tips and some great inspiration in these pages.

It doesn't take much to start to gain control of your life. You can do it a little piece at a time. Take the first story in Chapter 1, "Getting Started," as an example. Douglas Brown was 80 pounds overweight and was rejected when he applied for life insurance. This spurred him to action. He started simply—taking the stairs in his four-floor office building every day. Over time, this led to a complete change in his fitness and diet and he is a much happier and healthier guy today.

You really can learn to love exercise. In Chapter 2, "Exercise Can Be Fun," you'll read about Fran Signorino, who got in shape in the privacy of her home using my tapes. After a fairly aggressive perm, she even had my hair! And her family and friends tease her all the time when she says she is "doing Richard" and can't be disturbed. She says I'm always in a good mood and I make her keep trying even when she's tired. Happy to be of service!

One of the things I love about this book is that there are plenty of stories about "falling off the wagon." We all have our bad days, and that doesn't mean your diet and fitness program is over... it just means that you will do better the next day. In Chapter 3, "To Err Is Human," you'll read lots of stories from people who have their weak moments, including Rebecca Hill's very funny story about working on a fitness video shoot in Hawaii with a super fit staff. She was so embarrassed about ordering hamburgers from room service that she left the empty tray outside someone else's door every night!

Chapter 4 is about "Regaining Control" and you'll feel much better about your own slips as you read how other people got back on track. Kimberly Hutmacher describes how she has lost 20 pounds over the last couple of years in her story called "Resolution Not Revolution." She explains, "By keeping my goals small, I was able to follow through and sustain each one for the long haul." And in Chapter 5 you'll read about "The Gym" and how it really isn't as scary as you might think. Sally Schwartz Friedman has a great story called "Sweat Sisters" about going to a women-only gym where the social life and the great conversation distract her while she sweats her way to fitness.

You deserve to reach your target weight and get fit! And you deserve to have a *realistic* target weight. The stories in Chapter 6, "Liking Myself," are very important. The authors write about learning to like who they are and accept their body type. Some of them have struggled with too little weight and some with too much, but the key is to enjoy who you are and realize that you are beautiful inside and out, as Thurmeka Ward learns to do in her story about self-image called "Wonderfully Made."

One of my key themes is to laugh and have fun while you are taking care of yourself, and what better way to have fun than to have a diet and fitness buddy? In Chapter 7, "Having a Partner," friends and spouses work together to get in shape and strengthen not only their bodies, but their relationships as a result. Stefanie Wass describes how she and her husband walk every day to combat osteoperosis and how they are more connected than ever due to their daily time together.

Having a buddy can help you stay "accountable" too. I met a 402-pound man last December who is using me as his accountability buddy. Every week he sends me a journal of what he has eaten. He has lost 105 pounds so far in the eight months he has been doing this. In Chapter 8, "Telling Myself the Truth," you'll read about food journals and other methods people use to keep themselves honest. Sometimes we are not so honest, as Elizabeth Kelly confesses in her story, "Lying to Myself," when she discloses that she was not writing down everything she ate in her food journal.

You never know what will work for someone, and that's why this book includes a whole chapter on "Foods that Made a Difference." Bracha Goetz has a great story called "Soul Food" about how a friend reacquainted her with fruits and vegetables by discussing how wonderful apples are. This story had such an impact on the staff of Chicken Soup for the Soul that they are all eating apples now! Amy Newmark, who is the co-author and publisher of this book, told me that her mantra now is, "If I am not hungry enough to eat an apple, then I am not really hungry enough to eat."

You'll find additional great suggestions in Chapter 10, "Off the Beaten Path." One of these tricks may work for you. Jennifer Quasha describes how she has made a ritual of having a fancy decaf coffee each night while her young children eat dessert. She keeps a whole shelf full of different types of decaffeinated coffee beans and artificial sweeteners for variety.

Every morning I get up around 4:30 and say, "Thank you God for this beautiful day and I'll be kind to everyone in every way." Every day can be wonderful for you too. You can be proud of yourself and happy with the progress you are making toward your goals. Take an inventory of who you are and what you want, and then get started on the path toward "Shaping the New You." You're sure to find inspiration and companionship in these pages.

~Richard Simmons

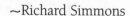

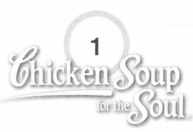

Through the Doors of Slimmons

My mother sold Coty cosmetics at Maison Blanche department store in New Orleans. Shirley was a delicious woman from head to toe. All four feet and six inches of her! Every day she would put on her four-inch high heels, fix her Grace Kelly hair and put on an adorable outfit. She knew how to do her make-up beautifully because she had been in show business. Sometimes I would watch her in the morning putting on her make-up before she went to work. In 10 minutes she could look absolutely gorgeous.

Well, in 1958 my mother won Salesperson of the Year, and the prize was an all-expenses-paid trip to Disneyland. I have to tell you, I was a Disney boy. My parents took my brother and me to every Disney movie that came out. And after the show was over I had memorized all the tunes from the movie. So when my mother came home with tickets in hand, I thought I was the luckiest kid in the world to be able to travel and meet Mickey in person.

I remember when we first landed at the Los Angeles airport. When I walked outside I immediately fell in love with the City of Angels. I looked up in the sky and I saw palm trees swaying in the breeze and the weather was unlike any place I had ever been. I grabbed Shirley's hand and said, "I am going to move out here some-day, Mom. I am going to be famous and I am going to buy you and

Dad anything that you want." And my mother looked at me and said, "I know you will, sweetie."

What can I say about Disneyland? It was an amazing experience. I rode every ride five times, except for the teacup ride, which I only rode once. All that spinning in the teacups made me turn a little green. We were there that day from 10:00 in the morning until 10:00 at night and I had to be dragged out of the park. I didn't want to leave the Magic Kingdom. I wanted to move into Cinderella's Castle. I got on both knees and I begged my parents to leave me there. I told them I would write often and let them know how I was doing. Days later I was back in New Orleans, feeling the heat of the city, but dreaming of California. I can't tell you how many years I wore my Mickey Mouse ears to bed. And in my bedroom hung posters that I got at Disneyland. Tinkerbelle take me away from all of this.

In 1973, I moved to Los Angeles. I did not know why at the time. I had no idea on earth what I wanted to do with my life. I had tried many careers, and I was good at my work, but there was something missing. I just knew that my career had to involve two things. One, it would have to be fun. I always had a quirky sense of humor and I spent my childhood laughing. Both of my parents were pretty hysterical. Two, it had to be a career where I could help people. My parents did a lot of charity work in New Orleans and they would take Lenny and me along with them to help out. And when we got home we would all talk about how good we felt inside for having helped those in need.

I remember the day I arrived in Los Angeles. I rented a car and checked into the Holiday Inn on Sunset Boulevard. The first couple of days I just drove around looking at the city. It scared me a bit. L.A. was so big. I drove through Beverly Hills and looked at all the mansions. I even thought, "Wouldn't it be nice if I could live here some day?" But then I just laughed it off.

Daydreaming is a wonderful thing, isn't it? I found a newsstand near the hotel and I bought a copy of *Variety*. I quickly found the want ads and went through them all. One ad really caught my eye. "Looking for a fun waiter and maitre d' to work in new chic Italian restaurant opening soon." I copied down the address, got in my car and drove right over to the restaurant. I sat there with the owners and gave them ten reasons why they should hire me. I did throw in a few Broadway tunes to make my presentation livelier. I got the job and I started work that evening.

Within weeks I learned how to mix a Caesar salad live and in person at the tables. And you know me, I went from table to table and made everyone feel welcome.

One day this lady came in to the restaurant and at the end of the meal she told me how much fun I was and how she enjoyed the food. She came back several times and brought friends with her. When I walked her to the door after she finished eating, she turned and said, "Pick up the Sunday *Los Angeles Times* and look under restaurant reviews, because I am writing about you and this dining experience." I stayed up all night.

At 5:15 a.m. I got the *L.A. Times* and with trembling hands I found the review. The headline read "Go See Richard." She praised the food, she talked about the baskets of French-fried zucchini and the veal topped with prosciutto, spinach and Fontina cheese. But most of the article was about *moi*. I read it with tears in my eyes. I could not believe she wrote all of those nice things about me.

From that day on, this little tiny restaurant with 12 tables became the hottest place in town. The phone did not stop ringing and some nights we served over 200 dinners. I would wear roller skates and roll around the restaurant. It was like one big party. I was having a ball meeting such fascinating people. The big difference about Los Angeles was that everyone looked healthy. They sort of had that "glow" to them.

While serving dinner I would always overhear them chatting about where they were taking exercise classes. I would write down the names of these places, because to tell you the truth, I had never, ever taken an exercise class. I was sort of a sickly kid. I had bad asthma and the flattest feet you have ever seen. And to top it all off, I was overweight. I never had to take a PE class because I always brought a doctor's excuse to school. I would watch the other kids exercise and think to myself, "Why on earth would they run around and get sweaty? I don't get it."

Both of my parents walked every day but I never followed in their footsteps. When my mother would turn on the TV and watch Jack LaLanne's program I got very upset. You see, I could not stand him. There he was, all tucked in to that baby blue jumpsuit. And he was always so perky. He would exercise to this organ music in the background. Who would ever think years later I would be a friend of Jack and Elaine LaLanne? I told him this story, and he gave me a big hug and almost cracked two of my ribs. He is still a very strong man and I love him so.

So with my list in hand, I took exercise classes all over the city. I took different kinds of dance classes like jazz and modern dance. I also tried Pilates and gymnastics. I went to several gyms in the city. And to tell you the truth, they just were not for me. All the classes I took were really serious. And what shocked me was I did not see one overweight person and everyone looked so perfect. I felt like the ugly duckling.

All the years before I came to Los Angeles I was a professional dieter and had never used exercise as a means to lose weight. Do you remember your first diet? I remember mine! It was the tuna, tomato, hard-boiled egg diet. Then there was the soup diet, the all protein diet. My mother would cut diets out of some of her women's magazines and slip them under my pillow. I must have tried fifteen diets by the age of nine. On these diets I lost only a few pounds. That is why I began taking diet pills that a girl gave me in school that belonged to her mother. I would take Ex-Lax. And when the weight loss numbers were still not big enough for me, I found myself falling into several eating disorders. I began throwing up and starving, which was so hard on my mind and body.

I knew I needed to start exercising. But there was really no place for me to go. The light bulb went off in my head. "I will open an exercise studio. I will open a place where people can come and sweat and have some fun." That was the day that I began saving all of my tip money. I put it all in a jar and would count it every week. When I was at work at the restaurant I began telling everyone about my plan to open up a studio. And they all said the same thing: "Let us know when it opens and we will come." I made real good tip money every night. But I had not saved enough to open up my own place.

One evening, one of my favorite customers came in. His name was David, and he was in the women's apparel business. I told him about my studio idea and he asked me how much money I had saved. He then asked me to come see him the next day at his office. He told me he believed in me and thought my idea was a good one. Then he took out his checkbook. I could not believe it. I did not know this gentleman all that well. But he wanted to help me open my place. "Go get them Richard, you are a nice guy. I will be there at the opening."

Well, I drove around and found this little warehouse that was located on a two-block street in Beverly Hills. I knew the first time I saw it that this was going to be my studio. My home away from home. It took several months for me to open and during that time I began to practice my moves. I would get all my records out and start choreographing to the music. I think I was a jukebox in my last life. I never missed *American Bandstand*. I memorized all the dances like the Jerk, the Twist, the Cha Cha, and the Monkey. I would play all of my records over and over again until I knew every beat of the music.

In the summer of 1974, I opened my exercise and motivational studio. I had a big opening. I invited everyone that I met at the restaurant. And who was the first person to walk into that studio? It was David, who made my dream come true. He proclaimed, "I knew you could do it, Richard, and I know you are going to be very successful."

From the day Slimmons opened it was a success. All the people who promised me that they would come showed up to sweat with me. And they told their friends and soon the studio was packed with people laughing and singing and sweatin'.

On Saturdays I began a class called "Project Me." It was a motivational and weight loss class. We would sit in a circle on the floor and talk about what we ate and how we felt about ourselves. I felt so good about that class. It gave people hope. Just like the hope my parents used to give others when they volunteered for their charity work. These people touched my soul. Many of them tried to lose weight the way I once tried to lose weight, but ended up feeling down and depressed.

I would sit there and teach them about food groups and about portions. I was teaching them my philosophy, which is "love yourself, move your buns and eat smaller portions of everything." Between the motivational classes and the exercise classes these people lost real pounds in a healthy way. They would run into the class and tell everyone how much weight they lost. And we would all applaud for their success. Their success motivated others to become successful too.

Slimmons has been open for 35 years. I am still there teaching exercise and self-esteem classes. Over these last 35 years, so many people have walked through the doors of Slimmons. Some of them had never taken an exercise class before, or it had been decades since they moved around. Hundreds of thousands of men and women of all ages, shapes and sizes have sweated with me. Many of these people were overweight and obese and had given up on themselves. But I could see a glimmer of hope in everyone's eyes. I did not just teach a class, I entertained them. Slimmons was my theater and they were the audience.

Once I put on the music everyone started dancing and forgot their troubles. While sweating, I would sing to them, laugh with them and sometimes cry with them. I saw their whole face change in a matter of minutes. I turned a lot of frowns upside down. They would all say the same thing to me. "I love coming here. I feel so alive, and when I leave I am always happier than when I came in." Their words just melted my heart. How honored I am to be America's clown and court jester.

What have I seen during all these years of leg lifts and jumping jacks? I have seen miracles. I have seen people turn their lives around. I gave people the tools to have better self-esteem and self-respect. I have seen individuals lose hundreds of pounds. Joyfully. And how does that make me feel? Like I am on top of the world! Over the years

I have been a good example to people. I have really sweated the sweat with them. I have always practiced what I preached.

Through the doors of Slimmons came so many people who believed in my crusade. Someone came in and asked me to be on a few local television programs. From there, I appeared on *Real People*. And then my big break came when I got to play myself on *General Hospital*. That led me to *The Richard Simmons Show*, *Here's Richard* and *Slim Cooking*. Through the doors of Slimmons came a gentleman who asked me to do exercise videos. And of course I said yes. That was 59 videos and DVDs ago.

I began writing cookbooks and motivational books to keep people going. And I began traveling all around the United States teaching classes like I taught at Slimmons. I became the Johnny Appleseed of health. I tell everyone in my audiences that they can lose weight and feel great and have a zip a dee doo dah attitude. I am still traveling today with my same message and the perkiness of Jack LaLanne. God bless him.

I hope one day you can come through the doors of Slimmons and let me motivate you. Or maybe I will meet you in an airport or you will come visit me when I teach a class in your city. I would be honored to meet you.

Thank you, Shirley and Leonard, for taking me to Disneyland and allowing me to dream.

Love,

Richard

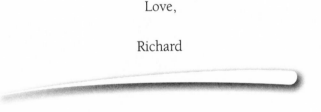

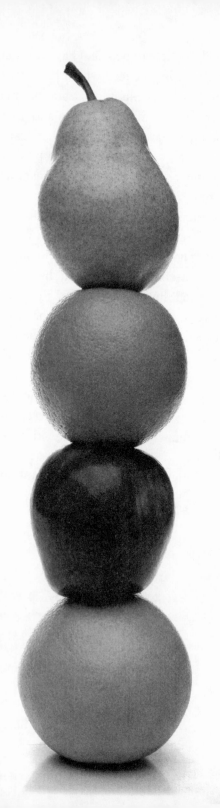

Shaping
the
New
You

Getting Started

*I am like a canvas
and the brush is in my hands.
Like the greatest of artists
I am going to create a brand new life.*

~*Richard Simmons*, The Book of Hope

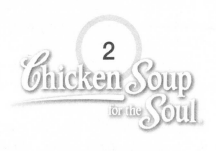

2

What Did I Have to Lose?

A man's health can be judged by which he takes two at a time —
pills or stairs.
~Joan Welsh

t started with my shirts. They didn't feel right. They were too tight and the buttons kept popping open. Buying pants with a 50-inch waist was a real downer for me too. Every time I put them on a hanger it reminded me of setting up a tent. But it was applying for life insurance that caught my attention and made me think deeply about my life and health.

I was forty-six years old and more than 80 pounds overweight when my employer offered a paid $250,000 life insurance policy for those who qualified. I got my medical records together and spent over $40 on copying fees. Three weeks later I got a letter from the insurance provider saying, "We have decided not to offer you life insurance." What it was really saying was "REJECTED!" I admit that being 255 pounds at 5'7" is not being in shape, but I didn't think I was that overweight. Now the insurance company was saying I was too risky because of my weight. Chances were I was going to die before age sixty-five.

I needed a lifestyle change, but I didn't know where to start. At the time, I thought exercise was the answer. I knew if I had to go to a gym, I would be faithful for only a few weeks. I had to do something that would not take too much time out of my day. I decided to start taking the stairs. Climbing stairs was a good way to exercise without going to a gym. I work in a four-story office building. Part of my job is going to other people's desks. I started my self-challenge. From then on, I would take the stairs.

The hardest thing was taking that first step. The first morning, I stepped into the stairwell and looked up. The three flights of stairs looked like Mt. Everest to me. Sir Hillary didn't conquer that mountain by staring at it. He had to take one step at a time. So I put my foot on the first step and pushed up, then a second step, then a third. Soon I was on the second floor, then the third floor. I made it to the fourth floor, wheezing and sweating and cursing myself for putting cupcakes ahead of my health.

I kept climbing stairs and soon I was up to twenty flights of stairs per day. Although my endurance increased and I started to feel more energetic, I didn't lose much weight. I then added a mile walk during my break time. That, too, helped my energy level, but I still weighed about the same.

About this time, I received a letter from my employer's insurance company stating that because my body mass index was so high, I could qualify for their weight loss management program. The insurance company would reimburse me for part of a gym membership or a weight loss program. After discussing it with my wife, I decided to enroll in a weight loss program. I studied different programs, and decided on one that was considered the most successful.

Then I received an e-mail announcing that the program I had chosen was going to meet in my office building every week. The e-mail invited everyone to an open house to see what the program was like. The next Wednesday, I went to the open house and liked what I learned. But I also learned that it would be $135 to start. I wanted to lose weight, but was afraid of committing my money. The group members were anxious for me to sign up. They needed at least twelve people to sign up, and I was the twelfth person. My wife convinced me to fork out the money and commit myself to make this weight loss work.

Because we met in my office building, I could attend almost every week. The instructor helped me to understand where weight comes from; it comes from eating without thinking. If I didn't keep track of what I ate, I ate a lot more. So I started writing down everything that went into my mouth. I also learned how to make healthy choices and read nutrition labels. We weighed ourselves every week and that helped me to stay on track. I knew if I indulged myself, the meeting leader would know about it next week. I also found the camaraderie helpful.

I began to see that eating properly was like sticking to a budget. I only had so many calories to use each day. I decided that junk food wasn't worth the price.

I began to see results almost immediately. I lost 10 pounds in the first three weeks. I stuck to a rate of losing about two pounds a week. After nine months I had lost 85 pounds and 14 inches off my waist line. People were amazed at the change. Some said I looked younger. I didn't think I was that overweight. Now I am shocked when I look at my old pictures.

I thought I couldn't lose weight. Thankfully, I was wrong. If you learn the principles of weight loss, and live those principles, you will lose the excess pounds. It takes work and discipline, but losing weight can be done. After all, what do you have to lose?

~Douglas M. Brown

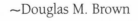

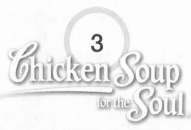

Video Exercising
for Beginners

Energy is that amazing feeling that comes to life inside of you
when you're happy and believe in yourself.
~Richard Simmons

I decided to go out and buy videos to help me exercise. I was too large and embarrassed to go to an exercise club to work out with a trainer. Besides, it was not in my budget. I was dieting and I was losing, but I needed to exercise. So I spent $6.99 each for two videos and I promised myself I would use them. They would not wind up on a shelf in the back of a closet.

My first choice was *15-Minute Workouts for Dummies*. I figured I had done no working out, working in, working up, or working down in over 20 years so I qualified as the Ultimate Dummy. Plus, the cover on the video said, "4 Easy-to-Follow Workouts." It sounded like a match made in Cellulite Heaven.

While video shopping, I also saw *Pilates Workout for Dummies*. I had seen many infomercials for Pilates that claimed to give the person doing Pilates a long lean body. I ignored the fact that I was barely 5'2" and would never be long and lean. The cover on the video also said, "An Easy-to-Follow Workout." If both videos were that easy, I could alternate them and pick my favorite for Sundays. I could even do both tapes on the same day and take Sunday off for good behavior. The added bonus was that both videos had nice smiling women on their covers and they seemed so fit! I could have tight buns and flat abs, too!

On Day One, I waited for my family to leave the house. There was no way I was going to do this in front of anyone. I got into loose shorts and a baggy top. Into the machine went *15-Minute Workouts for Dummies*. I listened intently as the woman with the cute red hairstyle and abs of Kryptonite told me to take my time and do fewer good repetitions instead of more bad repetitions. "I can do this," I thought to myself.

Then the music started pumping. It was Disco all over again, and the nightmare began. Instead of inhaling and exhaling to the pulsating, rhythmic music, I was hyperventilating. Within three minutes, I was winded. I could not keep up. I was reaching for my asthma inhaler. I was sweating. However, I kept my sense of humor. With my body still attempting to lunge and stretch with the super-fit Fitness Professional, being an adept multi-tasker, I picked up the phone and called my husband. (Heavy breathing.) "Sam, if I'm dead when you get home, please have them wash off the sweat, un-frizz my hair, do a tummy-tuck, and put me in my slinky black dress before you get rid of my body." He laughed and told me how proud he was of me for trying something new.

The truth was that not being able to do this video proved two things: 1) I was still the klutz I was in the days of Disco and 2) I was more out of shape than I had thought.

I worked through all four 15-minute workouts that day. I took long pauses and drank my water between each workout. They were good workouts. They were tough. I told myself I would never do them perfectly, but I would stay committed. After all, I had spent $6.99 on this video.

On Day Two, I did *Pilates Workout for Dummies*. It was a different type of exercise. At first, I liked it better because it was slower, but it was just as difficult. The stretching was easy to do incorrectly. To do it right took focus and more effort than I had imagined. I stuck with that video until the end. I rediscovered parts of my body. I hurt in places I did not want to remember. Then, I did not get up from the floor. I stayed on my back for about two hours. I earned a few hours of relaxation. If I was going to exercise, I was going to get rewards for doing it. I was even too tired to go into the kitchen. While stretched out on the floor, I realized I was tired, but I was NOT hungry.

That evening, I went to the closet where I hide things I don't want to find, and I found a gag gift my husband had received for his 40th birthday: *A Week with Raquel—7-Day Wake up and Shape-up Program*. On Day Three, I worked out with the absolutely stunning and incredibly fit Raquel Welch for 15 minutes. It was not a strenuous exercise. I looked at Raquel and thought about Raquel's body, wondering if it was like that because she always worked out or if she was just born that way. What Raquel did for me was warm me up for my Dummies exercises. I did not go all the way through the Dummies videos, but each day I increased the amount I could do.

Somewhere in the middle of this, I purchased two used copies of Richard Simmons' videos. I had always made fun of Richard Simmons because of his outrageous behavior, but I knew he offered good aerobic exercises for overweight people. I knew he spoke from experience and from the heart, and that is exactly what I needed.

His videos were actually fun. They were not difficult, although, again admitting how klutzy I am, I did not look quite as talented as the people who were *Sweatin' to the Oldies* with Richard Simmons. What I liked about his videos, besides the obvious upbeat music and easier format, was that the people who exercised with him were not all skin and bones. Some were full-figured. Some were even fat. In addition, at the end of the video, he introduced each exerciser and below their names, the total weight they had lost was listed. It gave me hope.

I decided a combination of these videos would be my exercise regime. I would work out and not get bored. If I did not like one video, but it was good for me, I would not have to repeat it for several days.

There was a larger benefit too. I was building up my stamina to attempt new challenges. When my husband and I both got home from work early enough, I was able to keep up with him on a walk.

This walk became an integral part of my exercise program, and was almost like going out on a date with my husband. We would walk and talk and be away from the phone, our kids, and our daily duties for an hour. Walking with my husband was fun.

I was also able to use light weights and those exercise gadgets I bought from infomercials over the years. They were no longer collecting dust or being used as temporary places to hang clothes I did not feel like putting in the closet.

What was most important was that I finally admitted that I was one of those overweight people who needed more to guide me back to good health. I needed more than diet. I needed more than supportive friends and family. I needed exercise, and I did not want to exercise with an audience. My video collection is helping me with that.

~Felice Prager

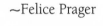

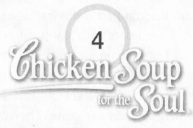

4

Taking Action

Movement is a medicine
for creating change in a person's physical, emotional,
and mental states.
~Carol Welch

"F at, female, and forty," the doctor said to me as I sat in his office. "I'm sorry but you fit all the criteria for having gallstones, and the ultrasound shows you have quite a few. That means you're going to need surgery."

Well, he couldn't have made it any plainer than that. I didn't mind the female part, but fat and forty? Didn't he know how many times I'd tried to lose weight? I'd drop 20 pounds and over time gain back 30. Disgusted with myself, I scheduled the surgery and left his office.

Three years later, I sat across from Dr. Eng while she explained her diagnoses. "You have acid reflux," she said, as she scribbled down a prescription.

"Here, this will block the acid," she said, handing me the slip of paper for the pharmacist. "You'll need to cut from your diet acidy foods like oranges, grapefruit, any of the citrus family. Also tomatoes, fried foods, coffee and tea...."

"Tea!"

"Yes, that only contributes to the problem. And avoid chocolate."

"No chocolate?"

My mind conjured images of rich, dark chocolate bars, chocolate cake, chocolate chip cookies, and Godiva hot chocolate, the drink I order when I visit the bookstore. Give up chocolate? She had to be joking. But the determined, matter-of-fact look on her face told me she was serious.

"Is there something else I can do to get rid of this?" I said, shaking my head and throwing up my hands.

"You could lose weight. As Americans get heavier, I see an increased number of patients who've developed this problem."

On the drive home, I considered what the doctor had said. I had battled weight my whole life. And I always lost the war. Now she was asking me to give up some of my favorite foods. I couldn't imagine life without the refreshing taste of oranges, tomatoes on my salad, and a cup of English breakfast tea, my morning ritual. And what about that bowl of chocolate ice cream at night? Chocolate, my favorite food.

However, according to the terrible churning in my gut and constant burn in my throat, I couldn't continue down the same path. And I had no intention of taking pills the rest of my life to remedy something within my control. Yes, it was time to act. But I had to be realistic. Knowing I'm not a gym girl, I needed a plan that I could stick with long-term. No more diets like in the past where I'd lose 20 pounds only to gain it back a year later. No, this time I had to do a complete lifestyle overhaul.

I made a mental list of the things I liked to do: read, write, paint, and walk. Walking, that was it. I'd start there since everything else on my list involved long periods of sitting. And I'd have to change my eating habits for good. That meant no snacking in front of the TV at night and then going to bed.

I took action that afternoon. When I arrived home, I said to our Bassett, "Come on, Charlie, we need to take our squatty bodies for a walk." He lifted his head from his comfortable corner of the couch and looked at me like, huh? We started out slow, and added a block or two each day. Now I walk up to two miles three times a week.

The next week I added a morning workout routine of crunches, leg raises, toe-touches, etc. Soon I built up enough stamina to do 20 minutes of exercise six days a week, in addition to my walking.

Sometimes, when I wake up exercise is the last thing I feel like doing. But I resist the urge to skip and force myself to do what I know benefits me. When I finish, I pat myself on the back for making the right choice.

I also took a hard look at what my daily diet consisted of and started viewing food as fuel for my brain and body. In a drastic move, I decided to stop eating all processed sugar and white flour for the first six weeks. This forced me to read labels on everything I ate, which at first made shopping take twice as long.

I became an expert at reading labels. As a result, I discovered high fructose corn syrup (HFC) hidden in many packaged foods. The syrupy substance lurked in our bread and even the clam chowder we had been buying. I also said farewell to frozen juices, most of which contain HFC. Instead, I buy the freshest in-season produce I can afford. I continue to read labels of new products because looks and packaging can be deceiving.

After the first two months, I treated myself to a small cone or dish of ice cream twice a month. After all, this is not a diet. I've retrained my thinking so I make healthier choices. Once I freed my body from the addiction to processed sugars, fruit and vegetables tasted sweeter than I'd realized.

If I do crave something sweet, which rarely happens now, I bite into a plump, tasty Medjool date or two. They halt the craving and I don't feel deprived. If I don't want a date, I treat myself to a dish of fresh or frozen berries, usually raspberries. Sometimes I still have two cookies, or a small piece of pie. But every day I make healthy food the priority, with an occasional sweet confection.

Sometimes, my husband and I stop for fast food when we're out, but I no longer order a regular burger. Instead I get a junior burger. If we get fries, we share a small package, and we carry water with us rather than buy pop.

The hardest habit for me to break was giving up my evening bowl of ice cream. One of the tricks I've used to conquer that craving is to floss and brush my teeth when I finish dinner. This signals my taste buds and my brain that we're done eating for the day.

The first two months, I lost 16 pounds. I still have a way to go to reach my goal. But I'm losing the weight with every healthy choice I make. Over three years I've managed to maintain a 35-pound weight loss. Three cheers for me. Not only do I feel better and have new clothes, I've also cured my acid reflux.

~Kathleen Kohler

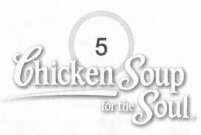

Right in My Own Backyard

If your dog is fat,
you're not getting enough exercise.
~Author Unknown

Obviously I needed to exercise more. I was overweight and in my mid-50s, certainly not getting any younger. Start walking, I was told. Everyone can walk, it doesn't require a machine, it's free, it puts little stress on aging bodies and what with iPods and cell phones one can almost put in a day's work while satisfying the body's need to move.

I began walking the dog and what a great thing it was. Except for that little problem of other dogs, of course. For while I leashed my Belgian Malinois in a strong harness and retractable leash, other dogs were running loose. The first one was a little Pomeranian who came running out on the street and bit my dog.

The Pomeranian lived, but I didn't sleep for three straight nights from the horror of it. Three months later it was a Cocker Spaniel. Amazingly, the Cocker lived, though it lost an eyeball.

"Some dogs just bring out the desire to conquer in other dogs," was how my vet explained it.

A few weeks later it was a Bichon Frise, just as cute a little dog as possible. The Bichon came running from her house. She did not attack Jo-Ann but it looked at first like she might.

I did spend a few weeks cursing the gods of careless dog owners, but when push came to shove the fact was that I simply could not walk my dog in my neighborhood any more.

It's hard to walk a dog when you can't take her on a public street. Walking the dog, however, became the least of my problems after I was diagnosed with very clogged arteries and needed a quadruple coronary bypass.

After my recovery a daily exercise routine became more than a nice diversion. In order to control impending diabetes and cholesterol buildup, I would have to exercise. Walking, my cardiologist told me. Walking is the best exercise for someone of your age! If you have a dog to walk, all the better!

I wondered about God's sense of humor and if He got the irony of it all.

As I recovered from the operation I would go out in the backyard and walk back and forth. The Belgian Malinois by then was not getting any daily exercise save her jaunts in the yard to do her business.

She joined me in my slow recovering walks across the yard and back and in due course I began to toss the ball around for her.

It began slowly but over time I created a happening morning exercise routine for human and dog in that backyard. I packed an old coffee can full of treats for Jo-Ann and every day I threw the ball and rewarded her with a biscuit when she dutifully brought it back to me. As my body healed, I took a slow jog around my "walking track." I started with one jog around, then two, on up to 10 jogs every day.

I took my morning coffee outside and sat it on the deck rail. With a piece of chalk I marked off my "revolutions" around the jogging track. To my and my husband's amusement, a perfectly circular area of bare ground appeared, my own personal jogging/walking track.

Indeed I put the leash on Jo-Ann, and after her ball fun and my morning jobs, walked around that track until I was up to 50 rounds each morning, one chalk hash mark drawn in for every five "circuits" around the track.

In the summer I hooked up a big box fan and sat a lawn chair in front. If it was too hot I could sit down and rest. Jo-Ann loved to play "tuggy toy" with me and that became part of our morning exercise fun.

Sometimes I will make all my phone calls on my cell as I walk around my track, sometimes I listen to my iPod, sometimes I record my "to do" list into the cell phone. When my granddaughter visits, she jumps out of bed in the morning and accompanies me around my track.

In spring I can smell the honeysuckle and watch the busy birds up close. Some mornings I bring out my kitchen scrap bucket and toss the compost pile with the handy pitchfork. In fall I rake the leaves, and this is also exercise.

I lost 40 pounds with this morning exercise routine and now I do not miss a day. The dog lost 15 pounds and the vet is overjoyed. I get up and do my morning chores, and after I gather my exercise bag, refill the coffee cup, and grab whatever gadget I might need for my morning plan. No machines needed, no fancy doodads, just a backyard, and best of all, no dogs unattended by thoughtless owners to terrorize me and my happy and healthy dog.

~Patricia Fish

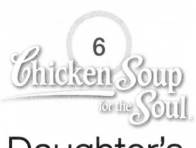

My Daughter's Gift

Action is the antidote to despair.
~Joan Baez

I was 5'2" and I weighed over 200 pounds. I never felt motivated to change my eating habits despite how uncomfortable simple activities like showering, dressing, walking, and even sitting eight hours a day at my job as a programmer had become.

I was in the doctor's office with my daughter, Amanda, when she was diagnosed with end-stage renal disease. The diagnosis presented a challenge I knew I would not turn away from. I was prepared to give her a kidney.

"Amanda, I can give you a kidney," I assured her confidently.

The nephrologist spoke slowly, not quite looking me in the eye. "Toni, you won't be considered a viable donor because of your weight."

Embarrassed, I glanced at my daughter.

"It's too dangerous anyway," she smiled, as she reached over and took my hand. "I don't want you to do it."

But her sweet acceptance of the situation made me even more determined. That day I made up my mind to lose the weight I had carried for more than 20 years.

"At work, there have been quite a few people who've lost weight going the low-carb route," I explained to Amanda as we discussed diet options. "Charles had success on Weight Watchers. Gail and her husband are on Nutrisystem. And there have been lots of positive results with Jenny Craig, Atkins, and the South Beach diet."

"You know," she cautioned, "you don't really do well when things are strictly regimented."

"Then I'll come up with my own version of a low-carb diet."

My diet consisted of the foods I liked the most and wouldn't tire of eating on a daily basis. Dinnertime staples consisted mainly of lean, braised steak or oven-baked shrimp and fish, with steamed vegetables completing the meal.

I eliminated all fast food, fried food and snack food. Bread, buns, rolls, donuts, muffins and potato chips were exorcised from the house, eliminating temptation. But by far the most difficult challenge was giving up Coca Cola. I never drank coffee, tea, water or milk. For years, the only beverage that passed through my lips was Coca Cola. Some days I'd down as many as four to six 20-ounce bottles.

Eventually I made new friends: Crystal Light, Nutri-Grain cereal bars, Healthy Choice and Lean Cuisine.

The pain of caffeine withdrawal overshadowed the hunger pains from my decreasing calorie intake. I counted calories religiously and as my daily calories declined my energy level increased. I remembered hearing somewhere that unless you feel hungry, you're not losing weight. As hungry as I constantly felt, I was sure I must be losing weight.

Keeping the big picture in mind, I weighed in only once a week and wasn't preoccupied with minor fluctuations. I didn't have a target weight or an end goal in mind when I began dieting. After all, I wasn't sure I'd even be able to maintain any sort of diet plan, but watching my daughter grow weaker every day gave me all the incentive I needed to stick with it.

It wasn't until I had lost 40 pounds that my co-workers, friends, and neighbors even noticed.

"Toni, did you get a new hairstyle?" my boss asked me one day. "It makes you look thinner."

That's one terrific hairstylist, I thought. Give her a big tip.

"How much weight did you lose?" asked my neighbor. "I told my wife it's got to be from walking the dog. I always see you out here."

That's a lot of shoe leather.

So I wasn't surprised when five new dogs became members of the neighborhood in the following months.

My slow walks around the block soon evolved into regular jogs throughout the subdivision, a pleasant surprise for our miniature greyhound.

"Are you sure you're not sick?" questioned my friends periodically.

No, I thought sadly, that's my daughter.

Months flew by and the diet became a way of life. Many of my cravings disappeared. Our days were filled with doctor appointments and medical testing to qualify my daughter for placement on the National Transplant wait list. No longer weighing in every week, I didn't even notice how much weight I had lost.

"I didn't even recognize you," gushed the nephrologist at one of our appointments. "I never thought you'd do it. How much have you lost?"

Hopping onto the scale in the corner of the exam room, I found I had lost 70 pounds.

I placed my arm around Amanda's shoulders pulling her close. "I think I'm ready to give my daughter a kidney now," I proudly informed the doctor.

"Finish her tests and once she's on the list you can begin your testing," instructed the doctor.

Finally the day arrived when my daughter took her place on the National Transplant wait list. And I was ready. I rushed to the LifeLink office on my lunch hour to fill out a mound of paperwork and begin the battery of tests required to become a living donor. First up, a simple blood test.

"We'll call you this afternoon with the results," said the donor coordinator as she walked me to the elevator.

Four hours later my phone rang. "What test is next on the list?" I practically yelled into the receiver. I was excited to get through all the red tape and get my daughter back on the road to health.

"Toni, I have some bad news." The coordinator hesitated a moment too long. "Your blood type is not a match."

My disappointment was nearly insurmountable. Instead of giving my daughter a kidney, she gave me the gift of a healthier life.

It's a gift I do not take lightly and will value forever, so I continue to count calories and count my blessings.

~Toni L. Martin

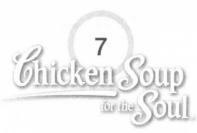

Diving In

Stand up to your obstacles and do something about them.
You will find that they haven't half the strength you think they have.
~Norman Vincent Peale

It took months for me to get the courage to go into the doctor, but I was at the point of desperation. I could barely walk. I sat in her office, heel throbbing, waiting for the painful blow. Whatever was wrong, I knew it had to do with the excess weight I was carrying and she would no doubt tell me to lose it. I was ready for her with the perfect excuse — how could I exercise being in so much pain?

After scribbling on my chart, she told me I had a case of plantar fasciitis. Though other factors caused it, it was exacerbated by being overweight, she said.

"It's hard to lose weight," I told her. "I can't really exercise with the pain."

"Are you eating balanced meals? Make sure you're not drinking your calories."

I assured her that I was doing my very best with food choices. Not exactly the truth, but I had been trying. I'd even seen a dietician for a couple of months.

"Try swimming," she said.

Excuse me? I must have misunderstood. She wanted me to put on a bathing suit and go into a public place? Forget it! Just because I felt like a whale didn't mean I needed to go put myself on display like some small-town version of Sea World. I left her office with a printout of some stretches and little hope of recovery.

A few weeks later, I could barely get out of bed in the morning. My husband and kids were doing virtually everything for me—I couldn't even lift 10 pounds without searing pain shooting through my heel. I decided that if I could get my life back, the humiliation would be worth it.

Early the next morning, I stood at the edge of the pool, feeling every bit like the Orcas that swam off the coast in my hometown on the Oregon Coast, except, could I remember how to swim? It had been years. As I edged in, bracing myself against the cold, I glanced at the lifeguard slouching in the chair; he was a skinny teenage boy. Thankfully, he didn't seem to be too alarmed to see such a big woman getting into the pool. I half-wondered if he'd be able to help me if I were to get into trouble.

As I started stroking over to the other side, a miraculous change occurred. Every extra pound seemed weightless. In the water, I could move gracefully. Though I huffed and puffed, the movement after months of inactivity invigorated me. I swam lap after lap for half an hour. For that little bit of time, I felt truly free in my movements, almost like flying. It was the only way to move without stabbing pain in my heel.

I started a three-times-a-week regimen and added laps each time, until I was swimming over a mile. It took 60 minutes, but it became my lifeline. I had lots of time to think as I propelled myself back and forth across the pool. "Being like an Orca isn't so bad," I thought. "They really are graceful animals."

Sometimes it was difficult to force myself out of bed so early in the morning to swim. After a few months, I noticed that I rarely had pain in my heel. The exercise improved my mental outlook on life; I was happier with myself and it became easier to make wise food choices. The best part was watching as the scale started moving downward! I was an athlete in a couch potato's body.

Now I swim, cycle, or walk on the treadmill five times a week. I continue to make progress, going faster and farther, all without pain. The scale continues to move downward, slowly but steadily. I still have a way to go, but I've been set free to regain a healthy and fit body.

~Lynetta Smith

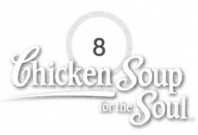

Doggone Excuses

> *Always do what you are afraid to do.*
> ~Ralph Waldo Emerson

I f there was a way to avoid exercise, I found it. Aerobics? Bad knees. Personal trainer? Too expensive. Treadmill? No room.

"There's one exercise I bet you can't dismiss," my husband challenged. "Walking. It's free, easy, and you don't need any special equipment."

But I had an excuse: fear.

I used to take walks. Lacing up my sneakers and hitching a leash to my spunky little spaniel's collar, we'd hit the pavement together. Kelly's tail waved like a banner, her nose lifted high taking in the mossy green scent of spring or the crisp autumn air. Walking with my dog, exercise was actually enjoyable.

Until one day when Kelly and I were strolling through a park adjoining my neighborhood. She wandered at the end of her leash along a bank that sloped down toward a river. Watching her curious exploration, I didn't notice anyone else around us until an alarming, hulking shape appeared: a dog big enough to eclipse the sun, ears flat, teeth bared.

I'm not usually afraid of dogs. But when I saw that huge, vicious-looking creature barreling straight toward us, I almost jumped in the river.

In the large, grassy openness there wasn't even a scrawny sapling to shield us. My grip tightened on Kelly's leash, my mind filled with fear that my pampered pooch would soon serve as an appetizer for the lunging behemoth. The dog bore down. I froze in terror. But Kelly yanked ahead, her fur standing on end all the way from her neck to the tip of her long, feathery tail. She wasn't afraid at all. She thought she could take that bad boy.

Then, in the distance, a young man wearing a hoodie sweatshirt whistled. The dog hesitated, turned and bolted back to its owner.

I was safely home in my easy chair before my breathing returned to normal. If dangerous dogs roamed the park, they could be anywhere. Loose dogs in the alleys, behind the railroad tracks. Even on my own street I'd noticed a burly dog dragging a broken length of chain. What about those stories of mistreated, mishandled fighting dogs? I lifted Kelly protectively onto my lap. "No more walks for us, girl." With that, I'd found an excuse to avoid exercise again.

Over the next few weeks I attempted a workout DVD, but plopped back down on the couch before working up a sweat. Those lithe ladies didn't inspire me to get moving. Before long my clothes started to feel tight again. While Kelly could run around in the backyard, that didn't solve my fitness needs. Maybe walking was the best exercise, but I was too afraid to face the prospect of another loose dog.

One Saturday as I sat working at my desk, Kelly lounged with her head propped up on the sofa arm, staring wistfully out the window. Was she missing the walks, the change of scenery, the enticing scents? I got up and joined her at the window. Neighborhood children scampered off a school bus. A woman with a stroller passed by. The scene didn't look as threatening as I imagined.

Day after day Kelly continued to stare, heaving heavy sighs, legs sprawled over the edge of the couch. I felt as lethargic as she looked. Although I didn't relish exercise, my body began to feel the effects of immobility. Heavy. Tired. Sluggish. I glanced at the door. Something in Kelly's deep, brown eyes urged me to get outside, for myself as much as for her. Maybe we'd try a short walk again.

Kelly jumped like a toy on a spring as I snapped on her leash. I looked up and down the street twice before venturing out the door. "Just one spin around the block," I said as Kelly marched beside me.

Peering between houses and behind parked cars, I listened for threatening snarls. White knuckles clenched the leash. This is no way to walk, I thought, ready to turn back. Kelly, however, trotted eagerly ahead, pulling me along behind her, unconcerned about what might lie around the corner. She wasn't letting that close call in the park prevent her from enjoying her walk. In fact, when we had encountered that huge dog she'd faced it bravely, ready to use whatever strength she had to run him off. Didn't I have at least as much might and courage as my fearless spaniel? I loosened my grip and moved ahead. Staying alert to my surroundings, I could spot a potential situation before a problem arose. If need be, I could change directions or cross the street. I even could grab my cell phone if I really needed help.

Then, from behind, I heard the scratching of paws on the pavement. A raspy snort; a menacing warning. Every muscle in my body tensed, my fear realized. A loose dog—coming right at us.

I spun around. The terrifying canine stood about ankle high. Long, caramel fur fell from a red bow on the top of its head, around its pushed-in nose and dainty ears. A little rhinestone-studded collar surrounded its neck. Four tiny paws scampered at our feet. "Yip!" it barked.

Fear quickly evaporated as I laughed out loud. Kelly casually sniffed the miniature dog. The pup gave one last yip and left, and we continued on our way.

When we got home I hung the leash in the hall, and Kelly stared up at me with her soft, wide eyes. "We'll go out again tomorrow," I promised, patting her head. Maybe I was still wary of loose dogs, but that wouldn't stop me from taking our walk. With exercise, just like in life, hurdles may appear larger than they truly are. And, although I may be expecting an obstacle the size of a Great Dane, often I find it's only the size of a Pomeranian.

~Peggy Frezon

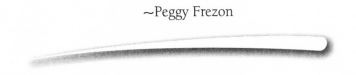

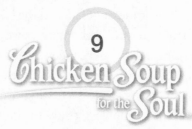

Saving Myself

A journey of a thousand miles begins with a single step.
~Lao Tzu

The nurse pulled off all the wires from the EKG machine, piled them back onto the cart, and moved toward the door. "The doctor will take a look at the strip and let you know. You can get dressed again." The nurse was gone with a click of the door. I quickly jumped off the table, and got dressed so I could feel less like a patient, and sat down on the chair to wait for the doctor. My chest began to tighten again and fear prickled my skin. It was hard to get in a breath because my lungs felt hard, like stone. I picked at my nails and tried to focus on pleasant thoughts but my mind kept playing the same distressing loop over and over again.

My symptoms had been persistent, but even worse, they were similar to my husband's right before he was diagnosed with congestive heart failure. I couldn't stop thinking the same thoughts of doom. How safe would our daughter feel if both her parents have a heart condition? I picked at my nails with more urgency. My husband now had a defibrillator in his chest, a clunky square that could be seen through his skin. He'd been afraid of it, and although I had said encouraging things about it prior to his surgery, I secretly didn't blame him one bit. He constantly feared it would malfunction, and he was stuck with it for the rest of his life. I was only in my 40s and I didn't want to have a weak heart or a box stuck into my chest.

The doctor returned, sat down on a stool and looked at my EKG strip. "This looks fine," he said. "Your problem is high blood pressure." I thought it over for a moment and then straightened up in my chair. I can fix high blood pressure, I thought. That's something I can change. After worrying for several weeks about my tight chest and breathing troubles, this seemed like a second chance. I didn't have a serious heart condition, there was no defibrillator in my immediate future, and I could ensure that it stayed that way. The doctor got out his prescription pad and began scribbling with his pen.

"I'm putting you on a medication to bring down your blood pressure," he said. I felt a little let down as I watched him write. I was hoping to do this without medication but I wasn't going to let it get me down.

"Do people ever get off these meds? I've heard that once you start on blood pressure meds you're stuck with them for life."

"Some people do get off them, and you'll have to make some changes like cutting out salt, take up exercise like walking, and losing weight." The doctor had a touch of skepticism in his voice. I figured he'd seen too many patients who wouldn't change their ways so I decided not to be one of them. This doctor was in for a surprise.

The first thing I did when I got home was to take out my date-book and mark the day. This would be the first day of my journey. I set a goal to lose 106 pounds and my motivation was the best I ever had—to save me and my heart from an early grave. My previous goals—to look good at the beach, to look good for the holidays, or to be able to buy nice clothes, had never worked, but now each pound lost would mean one less for my heart to work against. Then there would be 10 less, 20 less, 50 less, until I made my goal. Every evening I would open the date book and draw a heart in that day's square if I ate right and cut calories. That would mean a crash course in nutrition.

My next step was a trip to the grocery store. I intended to buy plenty of fresh vegetables and plan healthier meals. I realized how little I knew about nutrition, and as I wandered around the store I suddenly had the feeling of being lost in a sea of dietary ignorance. I was clueless about where to start or what to buy. After awhile I headed for the checkout with what I managed to find and then went home to get on my computer.

Over the following weeks and months I pored over nutrition information that I found on the Internet and in library books. I searched the websites of fast food restaurants so I would know ahead of time what the best, and worst, choices would be when we occasionally treated ourselves to a burger. As time went on I began to feel more and more informed, empowered, and even shocked by what I was learning.

Total denial had never worked before so I learned I could eat one Oreo cookie instead of eight, or half a bagel and save the other half for another day. I used less butter and more olive oil in cooking, bought whole wheat breads instead of white, and read labels before buying anything. I was learning more every day and the knowledge I was gaining made it easier to say "no" to temptations not-so-well-meaning people would put in my path. I now knew what bad things could be found in many innocent-looking food items and I was prepared to avoid them without remorse.

My last step was to work more exercise into my day so I went off to the high school track to do some walking. I started at a very modest 3/4 of a mile and over the weeks I worked up to two or three miles at least six days a week. Early on I felt a little frustrated, as if I was hauling a wagonload of bricks behind me, and I would wonder when the miles would pass more easily, but eventually those days faded away and I began to feel energetic, and victorious. Each quarter mile would pass faster and faster and when I neared the end of my walk I would keep adding extra laps. The possibility of success was becoming more real every day.

There was a time when just climbing stairs, or keeping up with other people as they walked, would leave me breathless. Things were changing and I saw that clearly one day when I had to go to my daughter's school for a conference with a teacher. I followed him through the long halls and then up a flight of stairs, and at the top I realized that not only was I still talking normally, but I also wasn't discreetly trying to cover up any gasping. There was no crazy pounding in my chest either and I became excited over the fact that I was getting healthy and fit.

The best thing I did for myself was to not buy a scale. I waited until visits to the doctor to get weighed so instead of watching my weight go down one agonizing pound at a time I could see my progress in great leaps. I saw losses of 10 to 15 pounds at a time and didn't live by the scale on a daily basis. It was far better for my morale, and occasional slip-ups got absorbed into the passage of time.

So far I've lost 80 pounds with 26 to go, but the most satisfying part of all this is how excited some people get over my success. Now they seek my advice and follow my lead when it comes to good nutrition and fitness. Success tastes sweeter than any cookie I ever ate in my life.

~Jeanne-Marie Poulin

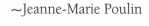

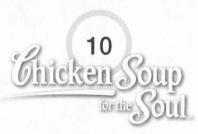

Fitting

Sometimes it's the smallest decisions that can change your life forever.
~Keri Russell

want to run away. There are more than 100 sports shoes lining two walls—it seems like every brand invented, every price imaginable. The staff at Frontrunners senses my hesitation. One asks if he can help. "I'm looking for running shoes." The words sound foreign, even though I've thought of nothing else for the past two weeks.

This sport scares and intrigues me. How can millions of people worldwide simply walk out their front doors and run? Where's the half-time show, the seventh inning stretch, the fights? Where's the fun in running past your neighbours, puffing like a train?

"I've never bought running shoes. Not serious ones that I wear only for running. I'm enrolled in a 10K training clinic and my goal's to run the entire thing," I confess to the salesman.

"All right. First I need you to slip off your thongs and roll up your pant legs."

What? I study his face. I came here to buy shoes, not flash my ankles. But he's serious, so I comply, wishing I'd taken the time to shave.

"Now stand on one leg."

I try not to stick out my tongue as I concentrate on balancing. Mental note: more Pilates for core stability. Jim assures me I'm not auditioning for the circus; he's looking at my arches to see how much they compress under pressure. He's also looking for pronation (inward rolling of the feet) or supination (outward rolling), though the latter is a rare find. Through a series of one-legged knee bends, Jim determines I'm an over-pronator; confirmed by the orthotics I wear.

Jim measures the length and width of my feet using a Brannock device. It is the only thing about this shoe-buying expedition that is familiar. My feet measure a size 8.5 and are a D width. I brace myself for the onslaught of men's shoes Jim will bring me. I hate trying to figure out which pair looks the least masculine. "Do you have a preference?" Jim motions to the women's shoes.

"My feet are too wide for those." I turn away from the softer colours.

"New Balance makes their shoes in multiple widths," he says. "I'll bring out a selection."

I can wear women's shoes? This is huge. I beam at the wall of pastel sneakers in front of me.

Jim disappears into the back. I glance at the price tags again. The cheapest pair is $35 for a pair of Adidas thongs. The most expensive pair is over $200. I've come prepared to spend between $85 and $150 for footwear, though the $200 pair look like they could run for me.

"It's a little tight here," I tell Jim, pointing to my baby toe.

He presents another pair. "These have a wider toe box."

I undo the shoes, pulling the laces as loose as I can. I don't want Jim to think I'll mistreat my shoes at home by kicking them off with the laces still tied. The pair he hands me feel like clouds. "I don't feel like I'm wearing anything."

"That's what you want. Wear them around."

I find myself hopping, skipping and striding around the clothes racks, trying to get the maximum amount of movement from each pair Jim hands me.

Finally, I narrow to two the ten pairs he's brought out. They both feel like my feet are floating and more importantly, they both look feminine. "I can't decide."

"Roll up your pants again," Jim says. I comply without hesitation this time. "Walk towards the door." He crouches, as he did when checking my arches and examines my gait in each pair. "Neither," he says. "You're still pronating too much."

It is then I decide to run barefoot. After all, it is what real runners seek to achieve. I'll reject this commercialism, and connect with the earth.

As a barefoot runner, I won't have athlete's foot, bunions, black toenails or hammer toe from non-breathing constrictive shoes. My soles will develop a thick layer of skin as they pound the pavement. I'll be like Barefoot Abebe, the Ethiopian runner, who won the men's marathon in the 1960 Rome Olympics. I'll be like the Tarahumara Indians running from village to village in Northern Mexico. I'll... I'll need a tetanus shot. Who knows what treats I'd step on running through Victoria's streets?

Jim has gone to confer with his supervisor. "The girl over there thinks she can run with rolling feet," I imagine him saying. "It's amazing she can walk."

I curse my ambition. Running the 10K seemed like a good idea two weeks ago. I curse my husband, Mike, who told me I needed actual running shoes if I was going to be a runner. Who cares if my cross-trainers hurt my legs after a jog around the block?

Okay, I do. Besides, my chiropractor said the same thing. "Running shoes are designed specifically for running because they are designed to move forwards and backwards, not sideways." So what am I supposed to do if Jim comes back empty-handed? I suppose that would be a sign to take up golf.

"These are the female version of the men's shoe." Jim presents the white and blue pair. I know the drill. I slide my feet in and Jim does up the laces. The shoes feel like a cloud, but I've been here before. "Now walk for me." He squats. Another salesman joins him; I've become an event. I walk towards the door, my pant legs rolled up. He's invested so much in me, I can't let him down. "How do they feel?" The salesmen grin.

"Fine." My voice is steady, but I feel like bursting. These are the ones.

"Great, let's box them up."

"Perfect." His buddy shakes Jim's hand like they've performed surgery and walks away. I sit on the bench, realizing I have no idea how much they cost.

Fortunately, $149.99 is in my budget. What I hadn't budgeted for was replacing the shoes in six months. "Are you joking?" I ask.

"Nope." He smiles. "Usually it's about every 400-600 miles if you're only running on them." I have to repeat this in six months? I should purchase all the New Balance 855s in Victoria.

• • •

There are 20 women in my learn-to-run group. Some of them, like me, are wearing new shoes with old leggings and long-sleeved T-shirts. Even though we only run for 30 seconds and walk for four minutes and 30 seconds, seven times, my face is red and I'm breathing heavily. But as we return to Cedar Hill Recreation Centre, I have never felt so alive.

~Alison Gunn

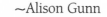

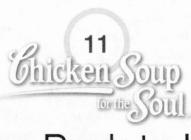

11

Walking Back to Health

Whether you think you can or think you can't — you are right.
~Henry Ford

I stared at my doctor in disbelief. I suspected what my mystery illness was, but now I had confirmation by a medical professional. I finally had a label. I was not crazy. There were millions of others, mostly women, who suffered the same way I did, with the same bizarre array of symptoms that I experienced day in and day out. I had fibromyalgia. According to the National Fibromyalgia Association, fibromyalgia is "a complex chronic pain illness that includes widespread pain, fatigue, sleep problems, and a variety of other issues, such as numbness, vision problems, stiff joints, and headaches." Although I believed I was predisposed for this condition, I began to have symptoms after two very difficult pregnancies. I almost bled to death after the birth of my second daughter.

I had an answer for what caused my symptoms. The question now was what to do about it. My doctor made it very clear. I could sit on the couch and complain about my pain and fatigue, or I could get up, no matter how much it hurt and do something about it. After prescribing medication for my pain and to help me sleep, he said the word that sends many people running straight for a bag of potato chips. "Exercise." How did he expect me to do that when every part of my body hurt? The truth was I had enjoyed exercising before all this had happened. Before my difficult pregnancies and the birth of my two daughters, I had walked diligently on our treadmill. I even belonged to a fitness center and worked out three times a week before

I was married. But that was when I was in my 20s. One husband and two kids later, I was staring at my approaching 40s and it wasn't looking so good.

There was one thing I knew for sure, and that was I didn't want to become a hurting couch potato. I wasn't interested in letting my medical condition get the better of me. I was going to get the better of it, even if it killed me! So I started out by returning to what was familiar, and that was walking on the treadmill.

I knew walking would help me and I could start out nice and slow. This was no time to start some new exercise program! I started by walking just 10 minutes a day, then added more minutes as I felt better. I figured if I didn't feel well, I could just get off. I needed to be kind to myself and listen closely to the messages my body was giving me. Any intense pain was like a big stop sign. But learning when to push myself was the hard part. If I stopped with any ache or pain, I would never progress. I had to learn the difference between temporary pain and pain that signaled injury. With fibromyalgia, this wasn't always easy.

While walking, I needed to think about something beside myself, to distract me from my discomfort. So I began to use my exercise time as a time of prayer. Instead of focusing on myself, I began to focus on others. Our treadmill was in a small room in our basement, so I posted prayer requests on the wall to the right of me, and Bible verses I wanted to memorize in front of me. This proved to be a wonderful distraction for me as well as getting me centered on the real Source of my strength.

Next on the agenda was losing weight. I had definitely put on pounds with my last pregnancy. I knew what I was supposed to do, having gone to Weight Watchers after the birth of my first daughter. But try as I might, I couldn't get myself to do the right thing. I would lose five pounds, and then put four back on. I was quickly going nowhere. I needed the accountability a formal group provided, along with admitting my need for help from God. Because my schedule had changed drastically with my two active, older daughters, going to meetings just wasn't going to work. So I looked into the Weight

Watchers online program, and it turned out to be exactly what I needed. Since I was already walking as exercise, reducing the amount I ate was easier. It wasn't easy, just easier. Changing your eating habits is never easy. It takes a solid commitment and a firm discipline to do the right thing. I also started praying about my weight loss efforts, for God to help me eat right and stay away from foods that were unhealthy for me.

The Weight Watchers program was a perfect fit for me. It teaches about correct serving size, and encourages eating more fruits and vegetables, along with providing a good tracking system to record these choices as you go through the day. It provided the accountability I needed. It was during this time that a friend told me about the benefits of drinking water. I learned that I was not drinking enough water throughout the day. This helped me tremendously.

Slowly I worked toward getting my health back. It was a long and difficult journey. Some days I would improve. Then I would have a bad day and everything seemed hopeless. But I kept going on. Having a positive attitude about my condition and believing that I could improve, with God's help, was one of the most important parts of my healing. If you believe you will never get better, you probably won't. But I paced myself, rested when I needed to, kept exercising, kept praying, and little by little, I started to see improvement. Slowly, I had more energy during the day, or my pain would be less severe. It wasn't overnight; it actually took about eight years. But I can do more now than I ever could before.

When I reached my goal weight, it really was a milestone. It helped me feel better and gave me momentum to keep going. Not carrying all that weight around helped lessen my pain as well. I even added a new form of exercise at that point: riding a bike. It helped to vary my exercise routine. And I was excited I could do something new!

I will never get rid of my fibromyalgia symptoms completely. I'm sure there will be times when they will worsen and then get better again. But one thing I do know, I will be prepared to deal with whatever comes. I will continue to eat right, and exercise. I will continue to have a positive attitude and to pray for others. And I know I can rely on God's strength to get me through.

~Joanna G. Wright

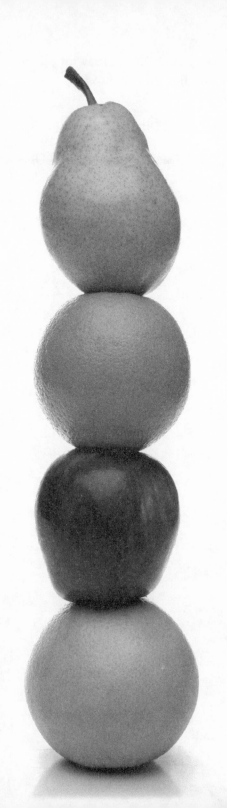

Chapter 2

Shaping the New You

Exercise Can Be Fun

*I will faithfully exercise
to stretch and strengthen my body
as I also strengthen my mind.*

~*Richard Simmons,* The Book of Hope

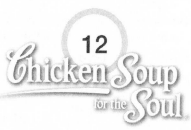

12

Richard and Me

The only reason I would take up jogging is so I could
hear heavy breathing again.

~Erma Bombeck

When I tell people that I've been "doing Richard" for more than 10 years, they look at me funny. My affair with Richard started the way many relationships begin — I was troubled and depressed. My parents had passed away within six months of each other. After that most stressful time, my blood pressure rose from normal to high. My doctor, believing that the condition was temporary, did not feel that I was a candidate for medication. He suggested instead that I exercise — preferably an aerobic exercise — of the low impact variety.

At that time, the last thing I felt like doing was jumping around. But because I am a lover of dance, I purchased a "swing along" with Richard Simmons tape and so began my daily encounters with him.

Richard's screaming and carrying-on irritated me somewhat on bad days, but his movements and "c'mon, get up — you can do it — I know you can" soon had me infatuated. Hey, you can't have everything in a relationship. On the plus side, I didn't have to travel back and forth to a gym; I didn't have to force myself to get up early to walk. I could meet him on both our terms. And in my own home. I quickly learned his routines as if I were appearing in a Broadway show. He was a steady and driving teacher.

I even got a perm during this period to save me time not fussing with my hair. Alas, it came out a little too curly, and lo and behold, now we looked alike. I had Richard Simmons' hair. Not by choice, but there he was looking back at me in the mirror.

The exercise outfits I bought brought me closer to his "look." My kids started calling me "Richard."

Within a month, my blood pressure stabilized, although my life did not. My daily workout with Richard helped me vent the stresses piling up each day. It was during one of these "workout" hours, intense on my part, that someone called me on the phone. I answered it, breathing heavily. "I can't talk now, I'm doing Richard."

"Scandalous," the caller replied.

Whenever I answered the phone totally out of breath, my callers would say, "I'll call you back—you're doing Richard." My son gave me a new workout tape for my birthday. He said, "New positions for you and Richard."

So now Richard and I could move while *Sweatin' to the Oldies*, and *Dance Your Pants Off!* while we were *Groovin' in the House*. And we got down with *Tonin' Downtown*. Richard and I went on company trips and vacations together. I brought Richard to the shore. He always wore the same clothes. We still had matching hairdos. Richard and I have been together longer than some of my past relationships.

I anticipate his every move and we mutually experience heavy breathing and sweating. This also beats some of my former relationships. Yes, I admit after all these years, I still "do Richard" and I'm now a grandmother. He's always there for me, he's always in a great mood, he always smiles and boy can he make the moves.

And judging from the assortment of tapes in the stores, it's been as good for him as it's been for me.

~Fran Signorino

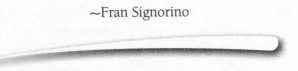

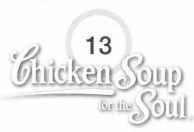

13

A Really Long Walk

Little by little one walks far.
~Peruvian Proverb

"Wow, the Golden Gate Bridge sure is pretty! And seeing it up close, through the fog — well, that's quintessential San Francisco, as far as I'm concerned. Whew, I'm tired. One foot in front of the other. Why am I doing this again?" My thoughts were jumbled as I climbed the hill through the Presidio. What was I doing here?

As a group of us made our way up and up, someone watching called out, "You're almost at the top of the hill. Once you get to that bend in the road up ahead... you can see the top from there." We groaned in unison. Still, we were nearly halfway done, I noticed, as we passed the 6- mile marker. Only 7.1 miles to go, I thought, until I walked across the finish line of my first half-marathon. In spite of my tiring legs, I smiled. I was really doing this. Two years of hard work were about to pay off.

Twenty-four months earlier, I found myself in a doctor's office for the first time in a number of years. I was nervous and anxious, yet there I was, waiting for my first physical exam as an adult at the age of thirty-two. But I knew what I would hear: I was overweight. Actually, obese would be more accurate. Getting on the scale and whispering to the nurse to keep moving the weight marker higher and higher was bad enough. But when I got my blood test results and learned that my cholesterol was sky high, I was angry. Mostly at myself, because I knew it was my fault, and that I was the one who had let things get so bad.

According to my body mass index (BMI), I was morbidly obese. And not only that, but my health was now at risk because my cholesterol was so high. I was running the very real risk of having a heart attack, and as a relatively young woman, that was awfully hard to accept. I had a decision to make: I could stay mad, or I could try to channel that anger into something useful. So I took a long, hard look at my lifestyle, and decided to make some serious changes.

Out the door went all of the high-fat indulgences that had become a regular part of my diet. And following them out the door was me, when I realized that I would have to combine dietary changes with exercise in order to lose weight. Walking was something I could do without a lot of preparation or expense, and so I walked. Short distances at first, just a mile or so, in jeans and sneakers. Within a few months, I had worked my way up to three miles at a time, and for my birthday, my parents bought me a pair of walking shoes. It was hard work, and I was completely overhauling my life. I paid attention to what I ate and read everything I could find about nutrition. I changed my sleeping habits so that I could wake up early and walk before I went to work every day. My life was changing, and I was changing, both mentally and physically. I had seen myself as someone who would always be overweight, but I was starting to see that it was possible to become a different (and hopefully better) version of me.

By the time I went back to the doctor six months later for a follow-up, I had lost 70 pounds. At my next physical a year after I'd started, my cholesterol was down to the normal range, and I was more than 100 pounds lighter. I was walking nearly every day, and I loved being active. I was doing things I'd never done before: hiking, biking, climbing a flight of stairs without feeling out of breath. As happy as I was with my new active lifestyle, though, I wanted to do more. I soon discovered that there were people out there who walked really long distances, and some of them even competed in races. And then I found it: a half-marathon to be held in San Francisco the following fall, two years after that fateful doctor's appointment.

Still, it seemed a little crazy: 13.1 miles? Me? I'd never challenged myself physically like that before. But if I had learned anything through this process, it was that having a goal which would be a stretch to reach could make me work harder than I ever had. So I started training that summer, and by October, I was on my way to San Francisco, nervous but also excited about the possibility of achieving something I wouldn't have dreamed of attempting just two years earlier.

I remember lots of random details about the race day: waiting in the dark for the starting gun to go off; the early miles as the sun rose; the big hill in the Presidio; my father cheering me on at the finish line. But mostly, what I remember is that despite the pain and the sweat, I was exhilarated. I had traveled a really long way during those past two years, and now I was doing something big: chasing away the fears that I would always be overweight, putting one foot in front of the other, and walking. All the way past the obstacles and the doubts in my head to a new, active, healthier me.

~Peggy James

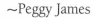

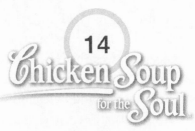

14

Fit for Life

Commit to be fit.
~Author Unknown

'd never given much thought to physical fitness. As a matter of fact, I'd never given much thought to exercise at all. I liked to take a walk, but I didn't go out every day or stick to any kind of schedule. I felt healthy, and thought I was in good enough shape not to have to do anything special. The idea of making a major life change to be physically fit wasn't very high on my list of essentials. It took being sidelined from the most basic physical activities to make me realize how being fit really affected my life.

The accident happened while I was out on a date. I'd wanted to go to a movie and sit and munch on popcorn and candy. She'd wanted to go roller skating together in the park. Skating we went. I hadn't been on roller skates in quite awhile, and I'd never been what you'd call a natural skater. I wobbled and flailed my way across the park on eight wheels, trying to keep up with the smooth, gliding movements of my date.

We had almost called it a day when she suggested we skate around the pavilion in the middle of the park. I thought it would be simple enough after trying to avoid runners, walkers, and park visitors on bicycles all day long. It was a simple little skate around the pavilion, a romantic moment that wouldn't take any skill at all. I didn't even see the pebble I tripped over. My right skate went in one direction, my left in another. The pain I felt when my right ankle twisted and popped was incredible.

I had to hop across a bridge and a baseball field and a parking lot to get back to my car. By the time we got to the emergency room I was red in the face, out of breath and in intense pain. The emergency room doctor told me I'd torn some ligaments on either side of my ankle and I'd have to be in a cast for three months. As I hobbled out of the emergency room on crutches, with sweat pouring down my face, I realized I was seriously out of shape.

If I thought that was bad then being on crutches for the next three months was even worse. I could barely walk 20 feet without wheezing and sweating and having to take a break. My weight shot up because I refused to move around much, and if I'd been offered the use of a wheelchair I would have gladly accepted it. But my doctor told me I needed the exercise to get back in shape and that my ankle would need toughening up once I was out of the cast. I retreated to my sofa at home and refused to budge from it.

Three months is a long time to be a hermit, and after a while I began to get cabin fever. By the time I went back to get the cast off my leg I was desperate to get back out into the real world. My doctor smiled at me when I told him I needed some serious rest and recreation and wrote me a simple prescription: Get Some Exercise.

I started by walking around the house. That got old fast so I ventured outside. Trips around the neighborhood offered me a chance to stretch my legs, but I knew I needed more of a challenge. The nature trails in a nearby park seemed daunting, and I only hobbled a few feet before I gave up. But it was springtime, and the sun shining through the trees beckoned me, so I forced myself back onto the trails and gritted my teeth through every painful step. I couldn't have cared less about how beautiful the wildflowers were or how the birdsong filled the air around me. I only wanted to finish my walk and go home to soak in Epsom salts.

Gradually, however, as the pain in my recovering ankle grew less, my resentment at having to endure these walks also faded. It was replaced by a slowly growing appreciation of the natural world around me, and the even more slowly growing sense of the physical wellbeing I was beginning to experience. I began to cover more ground with less panting, and after a while I was making my way through the foothills and park trails with ease.

I liked the feeling of fresh air pumping through my lungs and the muscles in my legs becoming taut and strong. I went in search of other trails. As I covered the natural boundaries of my town I branched out even farther and began to explore some serious hiking and climbing. I enrolled in a mountain climbing class, learned the basics of how to get myself up the face of a rock, and began to join climbing groups in my local area. Years rolled by. By the time I graduated to climbing El Capitan in Yosemite National Park, I was slim, trim, and filled with an energy I'd never had before.

A sprained ankle showed me what a little exercise and a chance to explore the natural beauty of our planet could be like. So now instead of a life of unfitness, I find that my walks, hikes, and climbs are making me fit for a life I never dreamed I could have.

~John P. Buentello

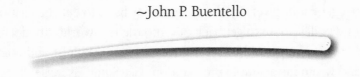

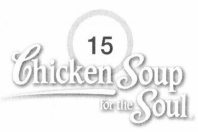

15

Competitive Yoga

Working hard becomes a habit, a serous kind of fun.
You get self-satisfaction from pushing yourself to the limit,
knowing that all the effort is going to pay off.
~Mary Lou Retton

I n my 40s, I started gaining weight. Not a lot, but the upward creep of the scale was inexorable, pound after pound, year after year. My clothes were tight, but I refused to buy a larger size. I'd gone up a size in my 30s after childbirth, and I wouldn't do it again.

When I hit my 47th birthday, I weighed just five pounds less than I'd weighed immediately before giving birth to an eight and a half pound baby. I had to start exercising. It was that or stop eating chocolate.

I have never been athletic. I couldn't even play kickball in grade school, and was the last one in the class chosen for any P.E. team. I'm competitive, but only at card games.

And I hate sweating.

Nevertheless, determined to lose the surplus poundage, I started going to a local fitness club near my home and tried out several classes.

I tripped over my feet during aerobics routines and Zumba.

Kickboxing brought out latent tendencies toward violence—I visualized punching out problem employees at work and recalcitrant family members, or the instructor who was inflicting so much pain on me.

Pilates wasn't bad, but was only offered once a week—not enough to stop the weight gain.

So I tried yoga. I didn't think my Type A personality was suited to yoga, but why not give it a shot?

The yoga instructor was an aging hippie who still dressed like it was the 1970s—tie-dyed T-shirts, sweatpants, and a leather headband to hold back her long graying hair.

The first time I went to yoga, my only goal was not to fall over. I stretched muscles I hadn't known existed. My joints popped when I twisted, and I wobbled when I tried to balance.

And I thought the meditation at the end was silly. Type As like me don't want to give their light and love away; we tend to keep them close to the vest.

"Namaste," we said as we bowed to the instructor at the end of class. What did that mean? The bowing was stupid. Why should I bow to a time-warped, style-challenged guru? But I followed form. I'm Catholic; I can do ritual.

The next time I went to yoga, I watched the other participants more than the instructor. I didn't want to look like a fool. If I was going to do this, I wanted to be good at it. I stuck my butt high in the air on "down dog." I set my expression strong and fierce on "warrior one." I couldn't get my foot up to my thigh on "tree" without hopping, but I could pretzel my arms into "eagle" with the best of them.

I knew my competitive approach to class was not aligned with yoga philosophy, but that conquering spirit kept me coming back. Damn it, I thought, I can learn this stuff.

In each class I picked someone to watch and tried to reach higher and stretch further than that person. My challenge was silent and secret. Over time, my furtive peeks at my classmates told me I was getting better. Well, sure, the gal in the front row could get her head down to her ankles on the "swan dive," and I was nowhere close, but she'd been doing yoga for 10 years and was still in her 20s. I knew I was as good as the other 40-somethings in the class, and my confidence grew. I was winning this game.

My smugness grew over the next few months as I continued my

one-sided competition. "Cobbler's pose" became as easy as "child's pose," my heels nestled close in my crotch while my knees stayed on the floor. I could overlap all four fingers behind my back in "cow's face," one hand stretching over my shoulder and the other coming up from my waist. My "tree" grew tall branches and sturdy roots.

One day I realized I was no longer watching my classmates. Instead, I was pushing myself to do better than I had during the last class. Could I stretch a half-inch farther? Could I hold the balance pose a few seconds longer? I was competing with myself. The bowing no longer bothered me; it was just another way to thank the instructor.

For the next several months, I worked zealously on self-improvement. I pushed myself in every class, and I improved even more—muscles stronger, tendons looser, balance more stable. I can't say that the pounds came off, but I felt good after class.

After about a year of yoga, I noticed my stretching was not even conscious, my poses more confident, and my balance came as much from my head as from squeezing my abs. Relaxation got easier. Maybe my mind was stretching along with my muscles.

"Namaste," I now say at the end of class, with reverence.

The salutation has many interpretations: "I bow to the divinity in you that is also in me," "I greet the God within," or "I honor the love, truth, light and peace in each of us."

Maybe I have an inkling what it means.

~Theresa Hupp

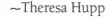

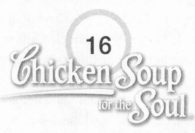

16

Raising the Bar

Sweat is the cologne of accomplishment.
~Heywood Hale Broun

Hanging from my sixteen-year-old son's doorway is one of those manly chin-up bars that brings out a guy's desire to continuously prove himself and his strength to others. My younger son bought it—with his own money—for his big brother this past Christmas and the two of them have since had countless contests. Since birth these boys have looked for ways to outdo one another.

Now—as the only female living in the house—I tend to just wander by their manly chin-up challenges, usually with an attempt at coaxing them into using their Herculean strength to help me—their mother—carry the huge piles of warm laundry from the dryer to the couch to be folded. Usually, they're too caught up in their own competition to notice me. That was until the other night when my younger son, Alec, grabbed my arm as I ambled by Billy's bedroom, which was beginning to smell like a sweaty gym sock.

"Let's see you do one pull-up, Mom," Alec grinned.

"Are you insane?" I laughed, knowing that I couldn't do one pull-up to save my life, much less my children's lives.

"Just one, Mom. We're not going to let you go until you do," Alec replied.

Both he and his brother stood tall, caging me in, their arms folded across their chests. I let out a huge sigh, knowing that I had to try. I reached up for the bar; this was not going to be pretty. As I hung from the bar, my arms quivering, I felt my eyeballs roll to the back of my head as I tried to pull myself up.

"At least try, Mom," Billy coached.

"I am trying!" I cried, sweat now beading on my brow.

The boys both laughed at me while I hung like a wet noodle from the bar; they encouraged me to jump into it if I had to. After what felt like a bad day at boot camp, I finally was able to get my chin up over the bar.

"You're going to do one every night until you get stronger," Alec insisted, as I slunk away in shame to my bedroom.

"Yeah, right!" I huffed.

The funny thing is, Alec has enforced that I do at least one chin-up every night and I am finding that it's getting easier and easier for me to pull myself up. What's even funnier is that I secretly do chin-ups during the day when the boys are at school, in hopes of really impressing them one day.

Oh, I doubt I'll ever get to the level of my kids, but it just goes to show that we are all capable of doing things we never would have believed we could do. With just a little bit of sweat and encouragement, anything is possible!

~Natalie June Reilly

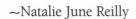

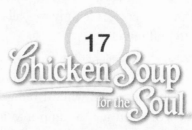

17

Life Changes

Your body is the baggage you must carry through life.
The more excess the baggage, the shorter the trip.
~Arnold H. Glasgow

"Dad," I said, via phone to Florida, "I've given away lots of Paul's stuff, kept the few things that we need to save, but don't have any idea where his car might be. Any ideas?"

While everyone else in the family had lived past ninety, my brother had managed to defeat his heredity by gaining over 50 pounds and dying of a heart attack at age fifty-seven. A pedestrian found Paul lying on a street in Skokie, Illinois near where he lived. I'd come to clean out his apartment and I couldn't find his car.

Dad suggested, "Look in the parking lot of the nearest Kentucky Fried Chicken."

It was there! I decided on the spot it was time to change my own diet. I wanted to emulate the long-lived members of my small tribe. Though I weighed only a few pounds more than I had in high school, the distribution of those pounds had shifted some... actually a bunch.

I was fifty-three, had been exercising moderately on a regular basis and eating a fairly reasonable mix of foodstuffs. I shifted to more fruits and vegetables and ate considerably less red meat. My wife, Lynnette, was a lifetime member of Weight Watchers—one of their success stories. She had *lots* of suggestions!

Two years later I was sitting in the cafeteria of a very large Air

Force hospital where I was a senior physician and overheard two nurses talking about the latest fad diet. One planned to lose 10 pounds before the holiday season. I remembered that the previous year she had gone on a different fad diet, lost 12 pounds and then gained 15 back. Then and there I invented my own lifetime diet.

When I got home that day I asked Lynnette to hear my ideas, partly to see if she was interested in trying the plan with me. I weighed 177, only three pounds more than usual, but that was well up from my college wrestling weight of 155 and my waistline measurement was three or four inches larger than I wanted.

"Here's my plan," I said. "Basically I'm going to eat less and do more, but I've come up with three ideas that form the centerpiece of the diet part of my regimen."

"I'm perfectly happy with my Weight Watchers plan," Lynnette said, "but tell me what your three ideas are."

"First, I'm abandoning the Clean Plate Club; I'll cut off a part of everything served to me and not eat it. Second, I need to quit snacking; I'm going to put our microwave popcorn container on the kitchen island with a bright red measuring cup on it and use that as a signal to STOP my frequent trips to the refrigerator. And third, I'll quit eating after supper even if we're at a party."

Twelve years have passed and I'm lighter than I've been since I was in eighth grade. When I see the red measuring cup, I say, "You Dummy!" and turn back at least 95 percent of the time; once in a while I eat some popcorn without butter or salt. I routinely pre-eat some fruit and cereal and then none of the goodies at parties.

As usual, I took things to extremes and started pushing my exercise, originally on a recumbent bike, later by hiking on mountain trails. Now that we're living in Fort Collins, Colorado at 5,190 feet, it's much easier to adapt to even higher altitudes. Recently, at age 68, I hiked up to 12,000 feet twice. I've got a third similar excursion planned with our friend Maggie, an accomplished mountain hiker, as my companion.

Next year I hope to hike one or more of Colorado's "14ers." We have 54 mountains that are over 14,000 feet high and 14 of those are rated as moderate hikes, ones I think I might be able to accomplish using good boots and hiking poles.

I'm working on next summer's expedition already. I've got a Base Camp with Lynnette and two friends, Maggie as our group leader and one other guy who wants to climb with us.

When I weighed 153.2 pounds one morning, under my intermediate goal of 155, I took a break from the diet and ate an appetizer, a full dinner meal, and a custard dessert at our favorite Thai restaurant. I've broken my diet plan into five-pound decrements, stick closely to my three ideas until I reach an intermediate goal, and then relax for a few days to a week.

Lynnette bought me a digital scale and I weigh myself every morning and keep a log of my progress. If I gain three pounds over a goal, I go back on the strict version of the diet; the weight melts off in a day or two.

My experience so invigorated me that I wanted to share it with others. I've started writing a short diet book, while Lynnette, who is the kind of cook who can fling together wonderful dishes from scratch, is adding the recipes.

Most people can't be as active as I am, but I've come up with suggestions for everyone. I park far away from stores, so I have a longer walk to get there. I hide the TV remote so I have to get up to change channels. And I'm deliberately absent-minded, so I make more trips upstairs to my den to get things.

As I neared the end of my first hike to 12,000 feet, I felt my brother climbing right beside me. I knew Paul would be glad to see how he'd changed my life.

~Peter D. Springberg, M.D.

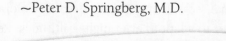

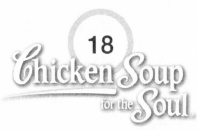

18

Dancing My Butt Off

There is a bit of insanity in dancing that does everybody a great deal of good.
~Edwin Denby

I don't know how it happened. Too much food, too much wine, too little exercise, middle age creeping up, surgical menopause... I am sure all of it combined and contributed to the 40 pounds I packed on over the years.

But it happened gradually and I didn't really notice until the day I stepped on the scale and realized that I weighed as much as I did when I gave birth to my daughter.

Of course, if I had been paying attention, I might have realized that the fact that I had about 30 pairs of jeans and 25 pairs didn't fit... yeah, that might have been a pretty good clue. But I wasn't paying attention to anything other than the fact that Spandex was my new best friend and I had developed cleavage!

It was time to make some changes. And since I was already making changes—my marriage was ending and I had decided to move halfway across the country—it seemed to be a good time to do something about my weight too.

But I wanted to be realistic. After all, I was in my 40s. And I had gone through menopause. Chances were, losing weight was not going to be as easy as it used to be. Chances were, I was going to have to work harder and get less results.

The first step was to sort through all those jeans. I had jeans in three sizes—8, 10, and 12. And I actually reached a point of fatness where I couldn't even get into the 12's unless they came equipped with user-friendly Spandex.

Repeating to myself over and over, "Be realistic. Be realistic. Be realistic," I sorted them into three categories: (1) I can wear these, (2) if I lose a few pounds I can wear these, and (3) there is no way I am ever going to get these zipped in this lifetime.

The day before I moved, I gave away a dozen pair of size-8 jeans that I was never going to be able to wear again. Most of them were like new—and I think some of them had never been worn at all!

That left me with 22 pairs of jeans in my closet—all 10's and 12's.

I moved. I started my new life, which included a new workout routine, a lot less wine, and healthier food. Admittedly, not having a husband to cook for made it a lot easier to just fix a quick salad for dinner. Not having my husband may have also made it easier to imbibe less alcohol but that's a story for another book....

For my workout routine, I didn't join a gym or buy a DVD. I simply did something that I knew I would enjoy enough to keep doing. I danced.

I put together an hour-long playlist of favorite songs to dance to (mostly classic rock and some upbeat country). I interspersed the dancing with a few spot-toning exercises and three miles on my stationary bike (which had doubled as a coat rack for much of the 15 years I had had the thing). And I was having fun! Every morning I cranked up the music and had a blast!

And you know what happened?

The weight started falling off. Apparently my metabolism didn't realize that I was older and menopausal. Suddenly, the size 12 jeans were way too big! Then the 10's got too big! And since I gave away all my size 8's, I had to go buy new jeans... because everything I owned looked like I was wearing someone else's clothes!

Four months and 32 pounds later, I seem to have stabilized. I am actually hoping that it's not a plateau because I don't want to lose any more weight. In fact I would like to have those last two pounds back... they came off my butt, which is now flat. My niece suggested I get some butt pads... I won't repeat what I suggested she do.

So now I am backing off a bit. Every other day I cut my workout routine down to half an hour. Occasionally I give myself a complete break and don't do anything at all! Interestingly enough, those seem to be the same days when I decide to treat myself to a chocolate cupcake and dish of my favorite ice cream. Steak for dinner. With a baked potato. A glass of wine. Or two. Oh, what the hell—I'll just have it all!

And then tomorrow, I will be back to dancing my butt off... literally.

~Linda Sabourin

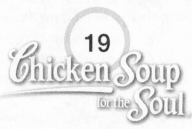

19

Commitment

We are what we repeatedly do.
Excellence, then, is not an act but a habit.
~Aristotle

It's 5:00 in the morning when the alarm sounds. I fumble the top of the clock in search of the off button, as the alarm rings in my ears. I roll out of bed and walk blindly through the dark into the bathroom. I flip on the light switch and put in my contacts. The house is still as I walk downstairs while my husband and three kids sleep peacefully. I lace up my shoes and take a deep breath. Some days I use the elliptical or go for a long run, but today I choose my favorite exercise DVD, *Insanity*. Sweat pours down my face and into my eyes. My heart races as I force my body to finish each exercise. As I near the end of the workout, my body's engine is now running on fumes, but a smile stretches across my face. It's not a smile because the DVD is over, but a smile of accomplishment from pushing my body to its extreme limit.

Some people are addicted to shopping, smoking, food, work, or even chocolate. But my addiction is exercise. Just like we need food and water to survive, I need exercise to get through each day. Some shake their heads when they see me run through town while hail pelts my face. Others get offended when I refuse to try just one bite of their grandmother's chocolate cake. They raise their eyebrows, surprised by my "no thank you," or by my choice to have a grilled chicken salad over a hamburger and French fries. Over the years, I have learned it's okay to just say "no." I shouldn't feel guilty for refusing food that I don't want to consume. It's okay if I choose premium fuel that delivers optimal results for my body. And it's my decision to, on occasion, indulge in a piece of dark chocolate or a treat without feeling guilty.

So what motivates me to roll out of bed to exercise at 5:00 a.m.? What gives me the confidence to just say no to ice cream? Commitment. A commitment to change my life with a solution that reduces daily stress, increases self-esteem and energy, prolongs life and above all improves my body shape. This is the point where a smile stretches across my face as I gaze into the mirror or try on my favorite pair of jeans that now fit just right. It's through dedication, commitment and relentless sweat that I can make a difference within myself inside and out.

~Sheri Plucker

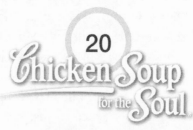

20

The Day My Metabolism Died

Take care of your body. It's the only place you have to live.
~Jim Rohn

When I hit thirty my metabolism went into a terminal nosedive. One week I was eating 16-inch pizzas by myself with no consequences. The next week I couldn't even lick a postage stamp without gaining two pounds.

First came the love handles. I'd always felt good about my midsection, never shying from removing my shirt at the beach. Then I hit thirty, and I treated my torso like a valuable family heirloom: I showed it to no one unless I absolutely trusted them, and even then I'd only bring it out on special occasions.

What had happened? The National Guard. I'd been in the National Guard for eight years, and so I had to run in order to stay in shape to pass the biannual Physical Training tests. Once I got out of the Guard, one of the first things I did was throw my running shoes in the Dumpster behind my house. No more running for me!

That's when my love handles, and their companion, my gut, showed up. So in order to get back into shape I bought another pair of running shoes and hit the streets. But there was one problem: I suddenly hated running.

Running was boring. Beforehand, I could imagine myself being deployed to a warzone and having to dodge bullets. Now the only thing I was trying to dodge was that annoying gut. Because I didn't have some short-term goal to shoot for, like passing a Physical Training Test, I kept finding excuses not to run.

But as I deluded myself, my belly grew. It had to be stopped. So I tried something drastic: Tae Kwon Do. I'd passed the sign many times while running, and when I peered in the window once to check it out, I saw 10 adults in white outfits kicking the air, or kicking targets held by the instructor, who I would come to know as Master Jung.

I forked over the cash and was immediately rewarded: the first hour-long class was brutal, full of painful stretches and cardio-revving kicks. At the end of the class we'd meditate, and when I got up the instructor would shoot me a look, as if to say, "Is that a pool of sweat from just sitting their cross-legged, or did you have an accident?" I was the only student who needed to wipe the mat every time I fell or sat down. I was like a giant snail, leaving a wet track wherever I went.

Having some financial difficulties, I could only stay enrolled in the class for three months. I lost 10 pounds. But more importantly, I learned an important fitness secret: find fun workouts. It's been years since I studied Tae Kwon Do. But instead of paying the monthly fee, I simply bought a heavy bag for $15 at a yard sale and hung it from a tree in my backyard. I practice all the kicks and exercises Master Jung taught me. And when I tire of that, I stop for a little while and rollerblade. And when I tire of that, I box for a little bit. And then there's basketball.

I've gotten myself back into shape more or less, if only a bit older. And rather than dread the prospect of running a few miles, I can roll out my exercise mat and get some frustration out on the heavy bag. When I tire of that, I'll go on to something else. There's always more fun to be had. I try to think of myself as a dog: If you throw a dog a Frisbee, he's not thinking about the exercise. He's having a blast. If you can trick yourself into having fun while exercising, you'll be more successful. So get out there, find something new, and have a blast.

~Ron Kaiser, Jr.

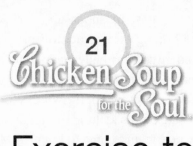

21

Taking Exercise to Heart

It is exercise alone that supports the spirits, and keeps the mind in vigor.
~Marcus Tullius Cicero

I was released from the heart unit of the local hospital the day after Christmas. It was my worst Christmas ever. With a throbbing headache and a hot water bottle on my head, I could hear my mother whispering to her friends on the telephone. A neighbor came to the door with a worried look carrying a casserole. She asked in a whisper, "What if she's disabled and not able to take care of the boys? Will you take care of all of them?"

Disabled? That was a possibility I'd never considered. What if I only came back from this crisis halfway?

Overweight and exhausted at forty-six, I was the single mother of teenaged twin sons. They took most of my time and energy. My career took the rest. My to-do list was always long and unfinished.

Additional tests the next day confirmed the symptoms were from too much stress. Though I only had borderline problems with high blood pressure and blood sugar, the message was clear: change my life now. Over the years, I'd gained nearly 40 pounds around the hips, waist and chest. That put me in the high-risk category for metabolic syndrome. I had to learn another way to manage my life and stress.

My lifestyle had been to come home from work, cook dinner, eat portions to match my athletic teenaged sons, and then go to bed early.

Exercise to me was as fun as bathing the cat. When I had physical education in high school, I thought of push-ups and running laps as punishment. I could never imagine exercising could be fun or a routine part of life.

That changed! Over my summer break, I met a friend who worked out regularly. Danica was active, shapely, and slender. This beautiful woman cooked healthy meals from basic fresh foods. She helped me learn to eat smaller portions and eat fewer desserts. Danica and I worked out with aerobic fitness programs four times a week. I began losing about two pounds a week, but more importantly, inches.

My sons and I always had several bicycles at home, as both of them raced in local bike events. I dusted my two-wheeler off and unsteadily rode it down the block. Then I started riding the bike to work about a mile and a half away. The tall fourteen-year-olds hooted with laughter at their wobbly bike-riding mom.

In time, I gained confidence and skill, and my wide behind began getting smaller. My big stomach was nearly gone.

Every week, I weighed myself and measured my bust, waist, and hips. Then I recorded the numbers on an index card. Wow! From 42-35-44 to 39-30-39. Seeing the results on the card helped me to say no to more food. By eating better and exercising, I was feeling and sleeping better and my posture as well as my attitude were better. I learned the more you exercise, the more you can eat. The sweets should be just a small portion though: one or two cookies, not six.

I still had not learned how to handle stress differently, but I would soon learn. Depressed one day, I went over to Danica's, not wanting to work out. I sat on the sofa staring at the wall.

She asked, "What's wrong?"

"Everything," I told her. "Today, I went to Virginia's to give her a birthday present, and she was labeling everything in her house so the kids know who gets what after she dies. She's having surgery in a week. What an attitude! Then I found out I am overdrawn in both of my checking accounts."

"Well," she said with a cheerful smile, "We're going to exercise and you'll feel better!"

I did. Through that, I learned that you exercise even when you don't feel like it.

Exercise had not just become a habit, it was a way to lift my mood, combat stress, stay flexible, and slow down aging.

~Jo Russell

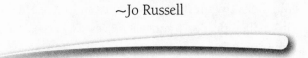

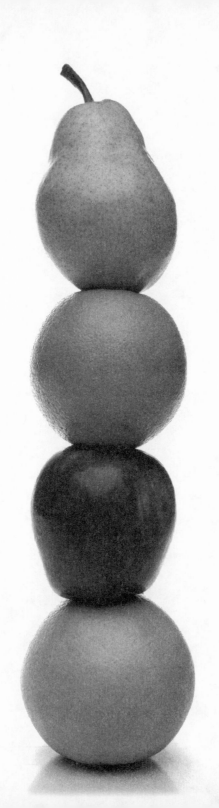

Shaping the New You

To Err Is Human

I will stop worrying about the past.
I will invest my energy in today
so tomorrow will be better.

~Richard Simmons, The Book of Hope

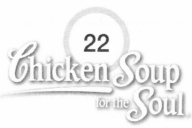

22

Cookie Chronicles

It's all right letting yourself go, as long as you can get yourself back.
~Mick Jagger

For 11 months I eat sensibly, but every December my willpower disappears. I stand by the oven like a child watching the minutes tick away on the timer. I anxiously await the first batch of gooey melted chocolate chip cookies and homemade peanut butter delights with crisscross patterns. I know if I indulge myself my belly will bulge and my pants will get snug. I eat them anyway. Not just two cookies with a cup of coffee, but two handfuls. And not just at breakfast or in the evening in front of the television, but for two full weeks, every time I pass the cookie jar.

At the end of a fun-filled Christmas Day, I dispense the leftover holiday cookies, cakes and pies to our four adult children and grandchildren.

"Take them with you. We're swearing off the sweets." Like the birds that return each spring with their melodious calls, I sing the same familiar tune as I vow to return to healthy eating: It's over; I'm finished; I mean it!

This December 27th I reached into the freezer and opened the box of veggie burgers. I removed one plastic-wrapped peanut butter cookie. I stashed the other five back under the patties. Guiltily I remembered my new mantra: "a moment on the lips, a lifetime on the hips." I decided to eat one for each hip, to even them out. I took my time and slowly nibbled my cookies. I knew the remaining four delectable delights wouldn't last much longer, so I planned to wean myself off them. I'd have one a day for four more days, then a new year—a new beginning.

I awoke hungry on January 1st, the other four cookies a fond memory. Time to reform and I meant it this time! I reached for the box of oatmeal—no sugar for me. I doused that pot of roughage with cinnamon, and sweetened it with blueberries. Right then and there, I vowed to start my antioxidant regimen and my exercise routine.

While my oatmeal was cooling, I decided to go for the gold; climb the flight of basement steps a couple of times, get my motor running, set my metabolism a notch higher, get a head start on the calories. I flew down the steps three times. No problem. The third ascent I dragged myself back up, huffing and puffing. I caught my breath, opened the cupboard door, but all of our cereal bowls were in the dishwasher. I reached to the back of the cabinet and snatched a faded, yellow plastic bowl. Three unwrapped chocolate chip cookies fell out. I salivated like one of Pavlov's dogs and stuffed an entire stale cookie in my mouth. My husband walked into the kitchen while I was on all fours. "What's for breakfast?" he asked.

"Shoatmeal," I mumbled with a mouthful of calories waiting to slide permanently towards my happily wagging tail end. I chewed frantically and considered tossing the remaining rock-hard cookies into the trash. But I couldn't do it. I decided coffee would make them palatable. After I ate that last cookie I vowed that would be the end. It was time to get on track. But I procrastinated and made excuses: The treadmill's in the basement and then I have to hike back up those stairs. The weather's too cold to walk outdoors. I don't have enough time to walk at the mall or recreation center before work, and I'm too tired after work.

As of this writing, my cookie stash is long depleted and I am starting to think about spring. Before I know it, I'll be ditching my comfy sweat suit and donning a new bathing suit. In anticipation of that purchase (it will be a size smaller, not a size larger) I have been taking baby steps towards my weight-loss goal of 10 pounds. Once I achieve that goal, I'll work on the other 10 pounds. I know better than to expect the thin me who lives within this chubby body to reappear like magic. It will take time to coax her out from all that padding. I've been padding myself with propaganda: A couple of cookies won't make a difference. Tomorrow you can exercise. Love the skin you're in. With age comes weight gain. Your butt's not THAT big.

The way I see it, at least from the rearview in my full-length mirror, my butt IS that big and carrying belly fat makes me look pregnant. If I attain my first weight-loss goal, I'll be ridding myself of this 10-pound baby I call Chubby. Then I'm going to work on his 10-pound twin, Blubber. These days, instead of sitting at work after I eat lunch, I walk. Instead of lying supine on the couch after I get home from work, I sit up and use a weighted flex ball to do leg lifts and arm exercises. I tune out my screaming knees and take those basement steps three times, twice a day. When I open the fridge, I pull out the gallon of milk and raise it over my head a few times. I dance the dinner dishes to the table; I high-step down the hall. When my hubby finds me on the floor, I'm not retrieving cookie contraband, I'm coaxing my body to bend and stretch. So what if I have to roll to get up? At least I'm working on my rolls.

I'm starting small; my goals are realistic. I may not hike a trail, but I am hiking myself off the sofa and I'm starting to move. My small steps are paying off. In less than five weeks, I've lost five cookie-pounds. Like the song birds that will be returning soon, I'm singing a new tune. And yes, this time I mean it!

~Linda O'Connell

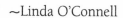

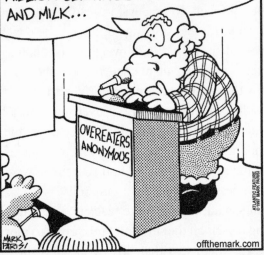

Reprinted by permission of Off the Mark
and Mark Parisi ©1997

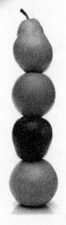

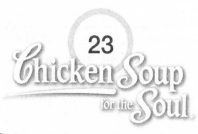

23

Cheeseburger in Paradise

You can't really be strong until you see a funny side to things.
~Ken Kesey

My name is Rebecca but my nickname is "C.B." which stands for cheeseburger. I got the nickname C.B. several years ago when I was working on a television show in Maui, which is gorgeous—just an absolute paradise! I was the personal assistant to ESPN television fitness star, Kiana Tom. We were in Maui for two weeks shooting her popular exercise show, *Kiana's Flex Appeal*. Let me tell you, two weeks is a long time to hang out with "fitness people," especially if your idea of a good time is a brownie sundae followed by salty potato chips. I was a bona fide junk food addict stranded on an island with "health nuts" who, from my perspective, seemed to be from another planet.

The entire cast and crew stayed at a luxurious resort called the Grand Wailea. The resort was expensive so we were required to share a hotel room with another member of the production team. My roommate's name was Julie and she was in charge of Kiana's wardrobe. (Kiana's wardrobe, by the way, consisted of itsy-bitsy bikinis and workout shorts. I always found it amusing that Julie's full-time job was taking care of bikinis that were so small I could have put three of them in my wallet!) Anyway, Julie was a fantastic roommate and I had a great time working on the show... except for when it came time for breakfast, lunch or dinner.

For breakfast everyone enthusiastically drank protein shakes or ate oatmeal while I desperately scanned the craft services table hoping for a doughnut that might have accidentally been delivered. There was never a doughnut to be found—the closest thing I could find was a whole wheat bagel. "Oh well" I thought, "at least it's the right shape!"

When we'd break for lunch, I'd watch in disbelief as everyone got excited about their grilled chicken breasts and steamed vegetables. I'd pick at my food claiming that I was "not that hungry." After we'd wrap for the evening, the cast and crew would make plans to go out to dinner together. Most nights I'd claim to be "exhausted from the sun" or say that I "had too much work to do" just so I could have a few hours to myself. I'd diligently work on my laptop as my roommate Julie got dressed to go out to dinner with the others, but the minute she'd leave the room I'd call room service and order a cheeseburger and fries. I'd salivate just waiting for the cheeseburger to be delivered! I was always struck by how high my room service bill was but it was a small price to pay for "real" food! I'd scarf down the cheeseburger in no time and then hide the evidence by walking my tray with the dirty dishes down the hall and putting it in front of someone else's hotel room door.

The production company had paid for our hotel rooms in advance but we were responsible for incidental charges like phone calls, in-room movies and room service so I figured I'd just quietly pay my room service bill at the end of my stay and no one would be the wiser. What I didn't realize was that this hotel offered a special feature where you could review your incidentals on the TV in your room. I also didn't realize that Julie would be checking our room's bill to see how expensive the phone calls she had been making to her husband had been. I was in the shower when I heard Julie yell, "$100 for cheeseburgers? That can't be right—I'm calling the front desk!"

I jumped out of the shower with soap still in my hair and said, "Wait. Actually, that's correct. I've been ordering cheeseburgers." I started laughing as I told Julie how I'd been ordering cheeseburgers from room service, then hiding the trays down the hall. She was laughing so hard when she called Kiana that she could barely speak. Then Kiana started laughing too and by the morning it had all become a big joke on the set. In a way it was a relief because it allowed me to eat my beloved junk food out in the open my last few days in Maui. As a matter of fact, on one of the last days of shooting I did go out to eat with the cast and crew. We were at a beautiful high-end restaurant so I ordered an exquisite pasta dish, but when my food came and the waiter lifted the fancy silver dome lid that was covering my food, it was revealed that someone had snuck out and gotten me a cheeseburger, then bribed the waiter to serve it to me instead of the pasta. Everyone laughed—especially me as I happily ate the cheeseburger!

Kiana still affectionately calls me C.B. but a lot has changed these days. I lost over 40 pounds through Weight Watchers and I recently became a circuit trainer at Curves gym. When new members say, "I just don't know if I can do this," I always reply, "Trust me. If I can do this, you can do this!" And when they ask for advice on what they should eat I hear myself saying things like "Oatmeal is good." And "For lunch and dinner you probably want to have some protein like grilled chicken or tofu, and be sure to eat your veggies!" At first they look at me like I'm from another planet but I know that will change. I'm living proof that with time and dedication new habits can be formed and taste buds can evolve. That doesn't mean that people suddenly become "perfect." I'm not. I still eat the occasional cheeseburger or doughnut but I'm more aware of my actions now than I used to be. It's still a struggle for me to stay away from fried foods and sweets but as I've grown older I've realized that everybody has challenges in their lives—food is mine. I take it day-by-day—sometimes hour-by-hour. And I'm okay with that because I'm proud of how far I've come since the day I got caught eating cheeseburgers in paradise!

~Rebecca Hill

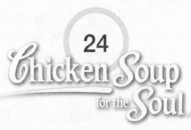

24

The Food Monster

I generally avoid temptation unless I can't resist it.
~Mae West

I thought I had killed it. I thought it was gone forever. For two years, five months, and 12 days (except at my son's wedding when I splurged on one small piece of chocolate wedding cake, three petite mouthfuls of fettuccine Alfredo, and seven glasses of expensive champagne) I thought it had left my body. It had lived within me for all of my adult life. It was probably there developing its sick sense of humor and evil personality from birth, but it wasn't until my adulthood that it finally showed itself to me. That's when I knew I had a Food Monster living within me.

Before discovering the success of a low carbohydrate lifestyle, my diets lasted a day or two at best, and, even then, I cheated. With terrible eating habits dating back to my youth, my weight soared and my body expanded. I was an overweight woman trying to hide inside oversized garments.

However, when I discovered the low carbohydrate eating style, I had not cheated. By keeping my carbohydrate intake down and my sugar intake low, I was always full and satisfied, and I was becoming thinner and healthier because of it. I had gone to office birthday parties, and while others ate birthday cake, I nibbled on a three-carbohydrate chocolate bar. My friends said things like, "I don't know how you do it!"

I knew my goal was more important than sugar-laden birthday cake. Out to dinner, I passed up warm bread and muffins, and I ate just meat and salad. I took pride in my strength and direction. A big treat for me was a piece of low carbohydrate cheesecake from a local restaurant or a handful of almonds eaten slowly over the period of several hours.

For the record, it had all been worth it. I lost more than 70 pounds and my goal was within reach. I looked so much better and could fit into fashionable clothes. I was motivated. I was driven. I wanted to be thin and fit and healthy.

Until yesterday! Yesterday, I needed a babysitter. Yesterday, I needed my arms tied behind my back. Yesterday, I needed duct tape on my mouth. Yesterday, I was bad.

The Food Monster who was hiding deep inside me finally showed its ugly face, a face I had not seen for a long time, but one that I immediately recognized and feared. I thought the Food Monster was gone, but it was just toying with me. It was playing games. It was lurking, waiting for my moment of weakness.

Yesterday was one of those days when I should have just gotten back in bed. Early in the morning, I was told my cat would need surgery to save his eyesight. I had gotten him to the vet too late, not knowing how dire his circumstances were. For several days, I had been putting medicine into his bad eye every hour on the hour in hopes that the eye could be saved. Yesterday I was told the cost of his surgery would be $2,200. I also discovered a leak in the roof over my garage, and the estimate for the repair of just the roof, not the inside painting, was several hundred dollars. I got my Visa bill, which included several visits to the veterinary eye specialist, one expensive car repair, and bills I didn't want to think about. When I got the mail there was a notice that I had been selected for jury duty. Yesterday was one of those days.

That's when I started making cookies for my husband to take to work. I had made 10 dozen of the same cookies a week earlier. My husband took the cookies to work, and the staff loved them. I think my husband loved them more than his staff since "there's never anything good to eat" in my carbohydrate-free kitchen. When I made those cookies last week, I did not even lick the cookie dough off my fingers. That is how well-behaved I was. It was so difficult, but I was perfect. I was so in control. Thus, I volunteered to make more cookies.

However, that was before my day started going from bad to terrible.

Unfortunately, in the middle of all the stress, I burned the first tray of cookies. Doesn't it just figure? Couldn't you have predicted that? I would not have burned anything if I were under the covers pretending to sleep.

That was when it happened.

Somewhere from the depths of my stressful day, the Food Monster surfaced with its evil laugh. It forced my hand to grab a hot cookie from the tray of burnt cookies, and it forced me to shove it into my mouth, burning my tongue and my palate. Then it made me chew. It made me chew fast. And then it forced me to swallow.

Mentally, I was unable to count the carbohydrates or the sugar that had just entered my system. Nowhere in my time on a low carbohydrate existence had I ever needed the carbohydrate count of homemade chocolate chip cookies, so I could not add it to my daily total. However, inside, I knew it was way over the top.

However, did this satisfy the Food Monster? No, it forced me to take another hot chocolate chip cookie, chew it, and swallow it.

I tried to rein it in, but the Food Monster was totally in control, and I was out of control. I had kept the Food Monster locked up for so long, but it was loose, forcing me to eat a third and then a fourth extremely hot, right-out-of-the-oven burnt chocolate chip cookie.

I was sweating and feeling remorse and guilt. Yet, until I found my inner strength, grabbed the tray of burnt cookies from the Food Monster, and dumped it into the trashcan, I was under its spell.

I sat down, drank several glasses of water, and tried to stop hyperventilating. I called two friends and my husband, and I admitted what the Food Monster had just forced me to do. All three told me that eating four cookies would not make me gain back the weight I had lost, but the guilt remained. My husband suggested I go for a brisk walk. He said the exercise would help me work off what the

Food Monster had forced me to do, and he said it would help alleviate the guilt I was feeling.

What the Food Monster did was remind me of just how easy it would be to lose control again and fall back into my old, bad habits. I love my low carbohydrate lifestyle. I love feeling attractive and feeling healthy. I love knowing I am in control.

However, yesterday I lost control. It reminded me that we who have had eating problems in the past will always live with them inside us.

Yesterday I went for my walk and did an extra 20 minutes on my exercise bike. The extra exercise did help relieve some of the guilt and helped me work off the extra carbohydrates. Then I mentally sent the Food Monster back to its cell, and I threw away the key once again. I know the Food Monster has an extra key hidden away, though, and I am sure there will be a time when the Food Monster uses it again. I will just have to be stronger and be ready to send it back to its cell when it does.

~Felice Prager

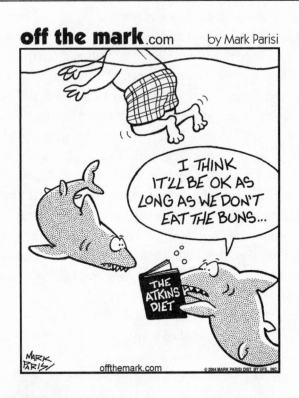

Reprinted by permission of Off the Mark
and Mark Parisi ©2004

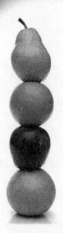

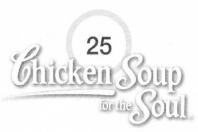

25

Playing to Lose

In every part and corner of our life,
to lose oneself is to be the gainer...
~Robert Louis Stevenson

After our first son married, my husband and I sat on the couch looking at the wedding photos. There were the bride and groom, barefoot and grinning as they stood in the grass. Here were the bridesmaids laughing and whispering behind bouquets of flowers. Another photo showed our son and his best friend toasting each other with a bottle of Jones Soda. And the next photo? A snapshot of myself with our guests.

That photo startled me. In my bright yellow mother-of-the-groom dress, I looked overweight. I felt embarrassed to have the photo appear in a family album. How could I have let myself get so overweight? There and then I resolved to get that weight off before the next family wedding came around with its photographic record of my image.

In college, I had been slender, but with the years, pounds began accumulating. They came slowly at first, but as I hit my fourth decade, in one six-month period I added 15 pounds to my frame. Still, the excess weight did not slow me down. Another decade passed before I took an honest look at that wedding photo and admitted the truth: I was obese.

After my son's wedding, I went to my doctor for my annual physical checkup. The doctor prodded me here and listened to me there. He smiled graciously and pronounced that I was in good health. Then, as he was collecting his folders and clipboard and heading for the door, I took the plunge and asked him, "What about my weight?"

Hadn't my doctor noticed that I was well above the weight limit for my height? Was my physician more willing to run the risk that I could die from a heart attack than risk that I might be offended?

"How can I get rid of these extra pounds?" I asked.

My doctor paused, set down his clipboard and, because I initiated this discussion about my weight, admitted his concerns. Offering several suggestions, he jotted down the name of a nutritionist.

Meet with a nutritionist? The idea intimidated me. I am a capable person. At work I solve problems. But now I needed someone to teach me how to fight a battle in a new arena. The nutritionist was understanding. She allowed me to cry and, yes, even grieve the loss of my favorite comfort foods. She assured me that I wouldn't be saying goodbye to those foods forever. I could still eat a chocolate brownie, butter a homemade sweet roll, or savor a piece of apple pie, just not all of them on the same day. Together we worked out a daily meal plan that suited my lifestyle.

Soon I was counting calories, comparing fats, and charting my carbs. Keeping track of all the numbers became a kind of game. I engaged my appetite as an opponent. As with any unfamiliar game, I had to learn new rules.

"I don't like cold foods. Raw carrots just don't do it for me," I complained.

My nutritionist suggested, "Lunches don't have to be the traditional salad filled with cold greens and celery. Instead, try cooking a plate of fresh hot veggies."

Why, I learned, I could even fix vegetables for breakfast! Vegetables for breakfast? All my time-worn rules about cereal and toast began to crumble.

My appetite, my unseen opponent, had lots of tricks to get me off track, but I was delighted when I won the game and stayed within my calorie limit for the day. Steadily the pounds disappeared.

But sometimes I didn't win.

Many years ago when I was a child, my grandmother taught me

to play cards. She said learning to play games was character-building: It taught children how to win and lose graciously. Thus, long before I learned to read, I played card games. As a toddler I learned to sort the cards into piles of red and black. Then I played simple matching games and memory games. And as I grew older, the rules became more complex and involved more strategy. I became hooked on games of solitaire like Canfield, Idiot's Delight, and Clock. Along the way I discovered that winning and losing is just part of the cycle of life.

In the same way, with my new eating plan, I found there were days when I won and other days when I gave in to cravings and tossed my diet to the wind. When that happened, however, I didn't give up. I might not win all the time, but I continued to play the game and develop new strategies in order to win the next day, strategies like substituting lower calorie items for my high-fat pleasures.

Three years later, I was no longer obese. By the time our daughter got married, I had shrunk six dress sizes. The photos in my daughter's wedding album show a petite bride radiant in her white gown while, standing nearby, her newly-slim mother looked on with pride.

~Emily Parke Chase

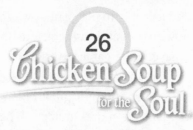

26

Brownie for Breakfast

Respect your efforts, respect yourself.
Self-respect leads to self-discipline.
When you have both firmly under your belt,
that's real power.
~Clint Eastwood

This morning I had a breakthrough. A breakthrough from the shame that had been a tremendous hurdle my entire life. Today I jumped over that hurdle. I jumped really high. And I landed on my feet. This time I didn't fall. This time I didn't even stumble.

Can you believe that I ate a double fudge chocolate brownie with milk chocolate frosting for breakfast? And it gets better. I ate it, I enjoyed every bite, and I didn't feel one ounce of guilt when I was finished. A piece of me had healed.

You see, when I was growing up, I felt ashamed whenever I ate anything sweet. "I see you sneaking that cookie," Dad would say with a glare in his eye. "You know what will happen if you eat those," he'd add. And I knew what he meant because he'd told me before. "That kind of junk makes you fat." My older brothers called me "Fat Pig." And I believed them. Granted I was chubby as a little girl, but technically I was never obese. But in my mind I just knew I was fat. Otherwise the people around me wouldn't have said so. And that was a problem. I was a problem.

If I even thought of eating anything sweet, I was breaking a law. At least my mind believed this lie. It led to a secretive obsession with food by the age of six. If I wanted something, I snuck it and ate it privately, or if I was in public, I'd eat quickly. I figured when I was finished, the people around me would be finished secretly criticizing me in their heads. Even at my birthday parties, I'd feel guilty for eating a piece of my own cake. I would pretend I was enjoying it and I'd smile for pictures, but negative thoughts bombarded me afterward: "Everyone knows your fat. You shouldn't have eaten that." Sometimes it would take days for those thoughts to fade. Some never did. Some followed me into adulthood. And it became a pattern that left me in bondage.

A five-year battle with bulimia intensified those negative thoughts. And I deprived myself of anything sweet even after I conquered bulimia so that I wouldn't have to punish myself afterward. Intense exercise and starvation were common if I slipped. Gaining weight was unacceptable.

I didn't understand that my struggle came from those unhealthy messages I received as a little girl. "If you eat sweets, you'll get fat." And "If you get fat, you'll be unlovable." All the unhealthy messages that I believed to be true were far from true. Being thin will not make people love me unconditionally. Just like being fat will not make people not love me. I deprived myself of sweets and/or binged on them in private my entire life and punished myself for doing so because as a child I was criticized for eating them.

Freedom came when I learned how to create healthy boundaries and how to take care of myself when I felt shame creeping in. Sometimes it just takes a positive thought to remind me that I'm okay. I can eat sweets in moderation when it's right for me and if I choose. And I can eat in peace because I know the truth. I deserve to enjoy my life. And to me, enjoying my life was having a double fudge chocolate brownie with milk chocolate frosting for breakfast this morning. Though I won't do this every day, I can do it once in a while knowing that shame and fear no longer exist in this area of my life. And I will celebrate self-acceptance and freedom as a reminder that being me is beautiful. That way, I will never forget it.

~Mimi Marie

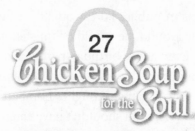

M&Ms Addict

It's better for food to go to waste than go to waist.
~Author unknown

There's a story that was jokingly told among my family. When we turned the couch cushions to do a good deep cleaning, there on my husband's side of the couch were a few coins, some loose change that had fallen out of his pockets.

"But Peg, look what's under your side of the couch," said my husband, Mike. "M&Ms!"

It was true. I was an M&Ms addict. I just loved those little chocolate candies. I loved the way they melted in my mouth. I loved the taste of the sweet chocolate. I loved the crunch of the candy coating. But what I didn't love was the way they contributed to my escalating weight.

M&Ms may not be diet food, but I considered them perfect in every other way. The flavors: plain, peanut, crunchy, dark chocolate, white chocolate, peanut butter, mint. And the colors! One of the best things to do with M&Ms was to sort them into piles—bright red, cheery yellow, dependable brown. And my favorite, gorgeous green. If only I could stop at sorting! But no, I had to pop them into my mouth. One, and then another, then… well, you can imagine what happened.

I can't say that M&Ms were totally to blame for my weight gain. Since my children were born, I struggled to shed my baby fat, anywhere from 10 to 40 extra pounds. I worked hard, exercised and kept the weight off for a while. Then I'd slip into my old habits and gradually feel my jeans' waistband tightening again.

If only I didn't have a sweet tooth. And if only M&Ms weren't so easy to eat. On the way home from work, I'd buy a pack to hold me over until dinner. At the movies — what better than a theater-size box of M&Ms? It wouldn't be so bad if I'd stuck to the fun size portions once in a while. But you know what's even more fun? The little candies come in 42-ounce, 56-ounce, and even 5-pound bags! Sometimes those bags of chocolate treats went on sale, and, you know it's never a good idea to pass up a sale.

So I'd pop some M&Ms in my mouth whenever I felt the need for a quick sugar fix. But the quick fix was becoming a big problem. How did I know it was a problem? Because I was starting to hide my M&Ms habit.

At first, I kept a regular-size bag of the candies in my pocketbook. I'd munch them alone in the car or at my desk, when no one was looking. Then, I hid a larger bag behind the spaghetti canister in the pantry. No one would notice its dwindling size as I made my way through the contents. When I was done, I scrunched up the bag and concealed it inside an empty yogurt container in the trashcan.

Meanwhile, my waistline continued to expand. I was cutting back in other areas, eating salads with low-fat dressing and skinless chicken breasts, but my candy munching was undermining the rest of my healthy eating.

One day Mike and I were strolling through the grocery store. We bought carrots and lettuce in the produce section. Then came the candy aisle. I paused at the tempting bags of M&Ms.

"Why do you like them so much?" Mike asked.

"They make me feel good."

"But food is just fuel," he said, "to nourish our bodies. That's all."

I frowned and slowly pushed the cart on past.

Over the next few weeks I began to do better at resisting my cravings. I ate rosy red apples when I wanted something sweet, a few almonds when I needed a crunch. And the weight started to come off.

Instead of sneaking sweets I walked the dog, knowing we were doing something healthy together. It started to feel good.

Then one day a package came in the mail. When my birthday arrived, Mike presented the beautifully wrapped box. "I ordered this before..." he said, his voice apologetic.

I ripped off the paper, opened the flaps and discovered the contents of the box. "Oh!" I gasped, holding up a clear, cellophane bag tied with a ribbon. Inside was a bevy of beautiful, perfect, M&Ms. All green. The kind you have to special order. The kind that are printed up just for you. I held them closer. Each one had words on it: "I love Peg."

"I understand if you don't want them," Mike said.

I beamed and hugged him tight. "Of course I want them!"

I put the candies in a pretty clear jar and tied the ribbon around the neck. I kept them on my countertop where I could see them every day. But I never ate a one.

Some things can make you feel good, without taking a single bite.

~Peggy Frezon

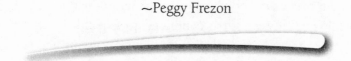

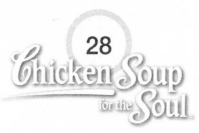

28

A Love Letter from Your Treadmill

An hour of basketball feels like 15 minutes.
An hour on a treadmill feels like a weekend in traffic school.
~David Walters

I see the way you look at me. Your head turns the other way as you walk by me on the way to the laundry room, hoping that I won't see the guilty look in your eyes as you pass me by. You never smile at me anymore. In fact, I hear you grunt when you pass me in the corner. And behind my back, you're telling all of your friends how much you hate me. You don't think I can hear you, but I can, and it hurts. You were on the phone last week, and I heard you say: "I know I need to get on the treadmill and start working out, but I just hate that thing. I just can't get motivated to start walking."

It wasn't always like that. When I was in the showroom, I watched you walk by and then return with a sparkle in your eye. You told the sales clerk that I was the one who was going to change your life. You said I was the perfect one for you. You had so many dreams, so many plans, and your new and improved life was going to start with me. You ran your fingers over my digital buttons and told the sales clerk that I was so sleek and so easy to use. And then you told him you had the perfect place in your home for me. Oh, those were the days, weren't they? You and I were a team. You needed me. You wanted me to be a part of your life. And now... well, now, I get a blank stare when you're in the room with me. You look at me as though I'm your enemy. I'm not your enemy. I haven't changed. You're the one who's decided you don't want me to be a part of your life.

I'm sorry that I'm whining. Maybe I'm being too hard on you. I guess you do use me once in a while—but for hanging your wet laundry. Didn't the sales clerk tell you that the dryers were in the appliance department? I'm a treadmill!

Listen, I'm not going to be bitter. I just want you to know that I miss you. I miss the way you look at me with adoration. I miss the way you tell everyone that you're going to spend time with me every day. Instead, I see you with the refrigerator. I'm trying not to be jealous, but I swear you have that door open at least a couple dozen times a day. You're always buying it sweets and treats. You always smile when you reach for ice cream in the freezer. I've overheard lots of loving sounds whenever you're near it.

I realize that you might have given up on me, but I want you to know that I'm not going to give up on you. I'm loyal, and I will be there for you whenever you're ready. I believe in you. I'm just asking a couple favors, though. Please don't talk about me behind my back anymore or give me the evil eye when you walk by. I'm not evil, and I think you know that. You're just not ready to let me into your life right now. I realize that it might take something deep inside you to bring us closer together, but while you're soul searching could you just stop by once in a while? You don't have stay long. Just let me know that you still care—about yourself.

I'll be here waiting for you. I'm not going anywhere.

~Heidi Krumenauer

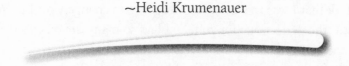

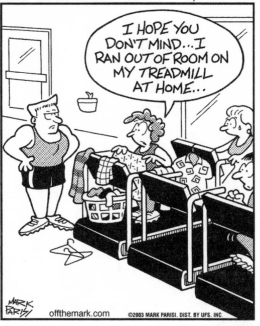

Reprinted by permission of Off the Mark
and Mark Parisi ©2003

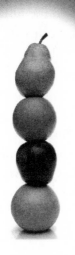

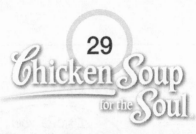

29

The Breakup

Strength is the ability to break a chocolate bar into four pieces
with your bare hands — and then eat just one of those pieces.
~Judith Viorst

My Love,

It is with the fondest regards that I am writing this letter. When I think of you, my heart skips a beat and my knees grow weak. I need you. I want you. I crave and long for you.

We've shared moments of sheer bliss when I've given myself to you. In the kitchen. On the couch. In my bedroom.

But my family and friends are starting to grow concerned. You've changed me. I do not like the person I see in the mirror. I've stopped going to the beach because I want you with me at all times and you can't stand the heat. I no longer enjoy shopping with my girlfriends because I can see you on every inch of my body and so can they. I cannot hide my love affair with you anymore because it is written all over my face. And my arms. And my thighs. And my abdomen.

Being with you has been great. The satisfaction I get from one night with you is unlike any other. Although, the regret and disappointment I now experience in the morning is increasing.

You've tried to tell me you're good for me in moderation but it never stays that way. One day turns into three. So much for moderation. You say I can see others, but no matter how hard I try, I compare everything to you.

I am writing this letter to you because I know that I am not strong enough to see you again. You are toxic and bad for me. I need a clean break. I cannot see you anymore no matter how hard you try to win me back. I know you are everywhere but I will be strong. Your alluring smell can no longer entice me. Your ability to know exactly what I want when I want it can no longer win me over. This is not going to be easy and I know I am going to miss you more than anything I've ever given up before. But I will be better for it in the end.

So, I am writing to you with passion, begging you to stay out of my life. We've had fun together but it's time I get over you. Goodbye, my love. Goodbye, chocolate.

~Christina Marie Harris

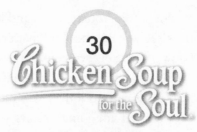

Guilty Steps

Every day I will find something to laugh about.
~*Richard Simmons,* The Book of Hope

In my on and off battle against the bulge, the bulge was winning to the tune of 20 pounds. Okay, 25 pounds. That didn't mean I was waving the white flag and giving up. No, I simply retreated to the couch with my honor guard, a six-pack of donuts, to decide on my next step.

Step? Of course, that was it. I'd walk myself thin. I would become, pardon the pun, a foot soldier in the battle against fat. And I would start immediately. Well, immediately after I finished eating my faithful troops. After all, I was going to need the energy for my walking.

To put my program on a scientific footing, I went out and bought an electronic pedometer, a device that counts every step you take. Now, as long as the batteries held up, I would have a daily record of my progress.

I even bought a calendar and a bright red pen to write down the number of steps I took each day. I put the calendar on the fridge where I would see it every time I opened the fridge. That way the calendar and I would be seeing a lot of each other.

Then I opened the package and took out my nifty pedometer. I felt healthier just holding it. Although the instructions were obviously written by someone whose first language wasn't English, I finally figured out which little red buttons to push to make the thing work.

I held my breath, sucked in my stomach, stretched out the waistband of my pants, and popped the gizmo on. I slowly released the waistband, hoping nothing would explode. But my pants and the gizmo looked fine.

So, I got off the couch and started walking around the house. Then I remembered to turn it on and started walking again.

Ten steps from the couch to the fridge, 12 steps from the couch to the bathroom, 25 steps from the couch to my bedroom. The fact that I kept using the couch as my reference point told me I hadn't bought the gadget a minute too soon. But as I watched those little numbers add up, I felt a surge of optimism.

This was going to be easier than I thought.

That night I put the pedometer next to my bed so I would remember to put it on as soon as I got up. The next morning I rolled out of bed, popped the gizmo on my pj's and started walking. Let's see, go to the bathroom, feed two cats, go upstairs, give third cat medicine, go back downstairs, walk to the closet and get clothes, get dressed, go back upstairs. Oops, run back downstairs, take gizmo off pj's and put it on pants.

By the end of the day I had logged 954 steps. By the end of the week my calendar was filled with little red numbers, each day showing a bigger total. I admit some of the increase was when I discovered I could have my cake and eat it too. Instead of sitting down to eat, I ate while walking around the house. By the way, don't try it with soup.

The more I ate, the higher my little red numbers went. I figured the steps canceled out the calories. The scale, however, took a different view.

Unfortunately, in the middle of the third week the cats found the pedometer on the night table. It took me two days and a lot of crawling around on my hands and knees before I finally found it under the couch hidden behind old candy wrappers, elastic bands and enough cat hair to knit another cat.

Based on the tiny teeth marks I found on it, I think the cats hoped it was food, then decided it was a toy. Or maybe they also tried the eat-and-walk program.

Although I felt I had gotten a lot of exercise crawling around, technically it wasn't walking. I wrote those two days off which meant two blank days on the calendar. I promised myself I would get right back on the bandwagon the next day and I did. And the day after that.

Then came the fateful day. I had every intention of walking, really I did, but it was raining outside and the couch looked so inviting and I was reading a good book and the cats all decided to sit on me.

One thing led to another, or in this case didn't lead anywhere. By the end of the day the number on the pedometer was so dismal that I didn't have the heart to write it on my calendar—I just left the square blank.

That was the beginning of the end. Every time I walked into the kitchen to look at the calendar and saw those blank squares, I felt a little pang of guilt which led to chocolate cake guilt, ice cream guilt and potato chip guilt. The guilt just got bigger and bigger and so did I. I finally realized I had to do something about the guilt or I would end up the size of my refrigerator.

I ripped the calendar off the fridge and went back to my couch.

All was not lost. I gave the pedometer to the cats who have been running and batting it all over the house and the numbers just keep growing and growing. I'm pretty sure two of them have lost a little weight.

You know something else? Now that I don't feel guilty, I've lost five pounds.

~Harriet Cooper

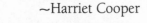

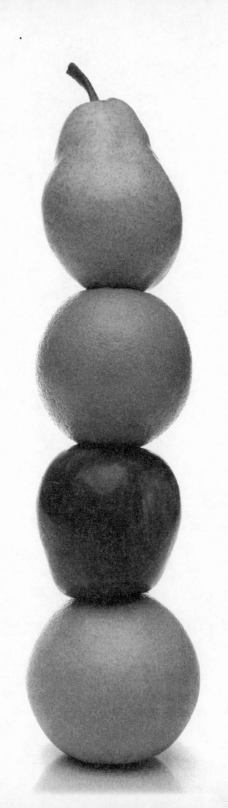

Shaping the New You

Regaining Control

I promise myself
I will not let one person,
one word, or one negative comment ruin even one second,
one minute,
or one hour
of my day.

~*Richard Simmons*, The Book of Hope

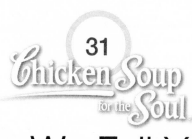

Are We Full Yet?

To the question of your life you are the answer,
and to the problems of your life you are the solution.
~Joe Cordare

I remember car trips when I'd ask my parents "Are we there yet?" over and over again. I also asked questions like "Why is the sky blue?" "Why can't dogs talk?" and "Why won't my little brother listen to me?" I asked dozens of questions each day, but the one question I never asked was "Are we full yet?"

There was no concept of "full" at our dinner table. My parents were young and doing their best to go to school, work and take care of two small children. My mom usually worked late so my dad was in charge of feeding us. He said we were to eat what was on our plate and that was that. My folks never asked me if I was full. Come to think of it, their parents probably never asked them if they were full either. As a matter of fact, I remember my grandmother telling me that she grew up in the Great Depression and there was never enough to eat at her house. She said it was a "privilege to always have good food" and that everyone should clean their plates. So we did—and not surprisingly, I never thought about if I was full. I didn't even know what "full" was.

When the concept of "being full" came up at my Weight Watchers meeting last year I stared blankly at my leader, Amy. "What exactly do you mean by 'full'?" one of my braver classmates asked. Amy explained that "full" means comfortable—a place where you're not hungry but you're also not uncomfortably stuffed. This brought up another issue. I'd never thought about if I was hungry. I didn't even know what "hungry" was. I simply ate what was on my plate when it was "time to eat" and that was that.

My classmates and I all looked at each other as if we were coming out of a spell. Most of us sat there dumbfounded while a few people began to speak. Many people shared the same story about being told that it was good to clean their plates. Others said, "Oh, so that's what people are doing when they put their fork down and stop eating even though there's still food left on their plate." I thought to myself, "Yeah, I remember seeing some of my friends put their forks down when there was still food. I thought they just had a lot of self-control—turns out they weren't doing anything consciously—they were just full so they stopped eating." Wow! Weird.

Over the next few months my Weight Watchers class continued to discuss the concept of being "hungry" and being "full" and I began to monitor myself. After months of practice, I could actually tell whether I was really hungry, a little bit hungry, full, stuffed or uncomfortably stuffed. Every time I ate I began to ask myself the question, "Are we full yet?" I started asking myself this every few minutes while I ate.

I've found that it's easy for me to tell when I'm full when I'm eating fruits, vegetables and whole grains. Things get trickier if I get into my "trigger foods" like cookies, cupcakes or potato chips. When I eat these "trigger foods" I have to decide on the appropriate (small) portion before I even start eating because my ability to detect "full" when I eat these foods is still out of whack. I'm a girl who can sit in the grocery store parking lot and eat a dozen cupcakes while swearing to myself that for some reason, "I'm just not full."

I really liked learning the concept of "hungry" and "full." It made me feel more in control. It is still strange for me to leave half my food on my plate or (on my good days) to pick at a piece of cheesecake and actually leave some of it on my plate. But I know I have to. I want to be healthy—and to be healthy I know I have to continue thinking about the quality of my food and when I'm full.

Learning the concept of "full" also helped me to get in touch with how different foods made me feel. For years I've been thinking that my Weight Watchers leaders Amy and Gwyndolyn were simply "toeing the party line" by pushing fruits, vegetables and whole grains. I lost over 40 pounds by following their advice but I must admit I'd roll my eyes when they extolled the joys of "delicious and amazing fresh fruit!"

I'm not a complete convert—but I have cleaned up my act a lot over the past few years because I noticed that when I eat a snack like an apple or a handful of almonds with skim milk I feel "full" as opposed to when I snack on say—half a sheet cake. The sheet cake doesn't make me feel "full"—it makes me feel crazed—and then in a heartbeat I go from "crazed" to nauseous.

The hardest part for me was detecting the difference between physical hunger and emotional hunger. Another Weight Watchers leader, Diane, brought clarity to me when she taught me about the "apple test." She said, "If you're not interested in eating an apple then you're not physically hungry." I often use the "apple test" to get a bead on if I'm trying to nourish my body or simply calm my soul. Again, I'm not saying I always make the right decisions (you'd know that if you saw the candy wrapper I'm currently hiding in the bottom of my purse). But at least I'm checking in with myself and trying to get in touch with my emotions and my relationship with food. I'm not perfect—and never will be—but I am much improved. I am interested in being healthy and I know the road to health is paved with fruits, vegetables and whole grains. I also know that a key to losing weight and maintaining weight loss is to ask "Are we full yet?"

Sometimes I still feel guilty about throwing food away, but my friend Nicole told me a great quote she heard—"Waste or waist." I like that—you can either waste your food by throwing it away or you can add that food to your waist when you eat more than you should.

This is tough stuff. A lot of it goes back to childhood. God bless our parents—they were good parents—who did everything they could to raise us right. But they never got me to ask the right question, the really important one—"Are we full yet?"

~Rebecca Hill

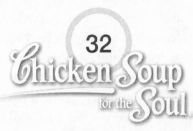

Empowered

Taking charge of your body can help you take charge of your life.
And that power can help you go wherever you want to go, every single day.
~Cheryl Bridges Treworgy,
member of five U.S. World Cross-Country teams

"Y ou've got to be kidding," I hissed through clenched teeth as I tried to put on my favorite pair of pants. I lay on the bed, sucked in my stomach, pulled and tugged, but the zipper wouldn't close. In disgust, I tugged them off and threw them to the back of the closet. I fished out a long wraparound skirt and tied it around my middle, then joined my husband downstairs.

"You look nice," my husband said.

"No, I don't," I shot back. "I'm fat." I caught a glimpse of myself in the hallway mirror. I didn't like the person I saw. How did I get this way? The weight started creeping on after the kids were born. But they were in their 30s now! A few pounds here, a few pounds there, and the scale continued to climb higher each year.

The problem was I hated the word "diet." To me it meant depriving myself of every good thing I loved. Even more I hated the thought of saying "I can't" every time I wanted something.

Later that summer, I found myself out of breath when I climbed two flights of stairs. And then, on a moderate hike with my grandsons, my heart started pounding heavily. I made an appointment to see my doctor.

"Your blood pressure is too high," she said. "You need to bring it down." Heart disease ran in my family, and feeling winded after mild exertion was a warning sign. "You're not that overweight," she continued, "but if you lost 15-20 pounds it would make a big difference."

Easy for her to say, I thought when I got back in the car and headed for home. Up ahead I saw the bright yellow arches of McDonald's. I pulled in. There was nothing like a juicy cheeseburger, fries and a shake to take away the sting of the doctor's warning. The next morning I stepped on the scale. I weighed more than I ever had in my life.

The next week I met a girlfriend at my favorite restaurant for lunch. All morning my mouth had been watering for the cheesy broccoli soup, grilled pastrami sandwich, and French fries. But I couldn't have any of it. "I'm tired of denying myself," I complained to my friend. "I can't have cake, ice cream, fries. Is there anything I can have?"

"You can have lots of things," she said.

"Yeah, right. You're not the one trying to lose weight." I sulked in my chair and thought about how I stepped on the scale every morning and peeked at the numbers. I was happy if I hadn't gained and elated if I'd lost even half a pound. I closed my eyes for a few seconds. When I opened them, my thoughts were finally clear. There was something I could have. Control. Control over my own decisions. I could pick something I knew would be good for me, or I could pick something that wasn't in line with my goals. It was all a matter of choice.

I closed my menu and plopped it down on the end of the table. "I'm choosing the Chinese chicken salad with the dressing on the side," I said to the waitress when she took our order.

I felt great when I left the restaurant carrying a take-home box filled with half of that huge salad. But most of all, I discovered I had control over my choices. I loved the feeling of power it gave me.

The weight came off slowly, but after a while it stalled. Eating a light meal a couple of nights a week would help, but that would mean preparing two separate dinners. My husband hadn't said anything about the changes I'd made, but I had a feeling he was going to say something about this one.

"What are you doing now?" he asked when he saw me bring a bowl of oatmeal to the table. He sat with a sizzling steak and a steaming baked potato. "You're not going to try to make me eat like that, are you?"

"Honey, I'm not going to change what I make you for dinner," I said. "Two or three times a week I'm going to have a bowl of cereal with fruit, or some healthy soup, or even oatmeal like this. I like those things. They satisfy me."

"But you'll get sick if you don't eat more. It's not good for you."

"It's all healthy food. And besides, I usually have tuna for lunch with crackers and carrot and celery sticks. Sometimes I have yogurt with sliced strawberries. I eat fine, I really do."

"Well, it doesn't look like it to me," he frowned.

Later that night, we talked. "I'm doing this to feel better about myself," I said. "I can't go back to the way I was. I won't. But it hurts when you don't support me in what I'm trying to do."

He took my hand in his. "I'm sorry," he said. "I didn't mean to undermine your efforts. To me, you've always been beautiful."

"You're sweet, but I'd appreciate it if you wouldn't comment on what I eat. It would help me a lot."

"Okay, if that's what you want."

And by gosh, he stuck to his word. I continued to make his favorite meals and he uttered not one sound. It was just what I needed to keep working toward my weight loss goal.

I added exercise by dusting off the old bike in the garage and peddling for 30 minutes after dinner. And I continued to make changes. A nice sized salad accompanied almost every meal I made. A little cheese on top or a chopped hard-boiled egg made it look visually appealing. "I love your salads," my husband said while rinsing the dinner dishes one night. He dried his hands on a towel. "You really look great," he added as he put his arms around me.

"Thanks," I said. Just that morning I'd tried on my favorite pants again. They fit perfectly.

A year later I was in the doctor's office for a checkup. I'd lost 15 pounds. She confirmed that my blood pressure was normal. Two years later, I've still kept off the weight. I like how I look in the mirror, but more so how I feel on the inside. No more "I can't" talk for me. I can lose weight, and keep it off. With the power that comes from wise choices, I know I'll have no trouble sticking to the lifestyle I choose.

~B.J. Taylor

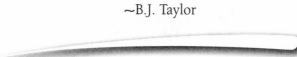

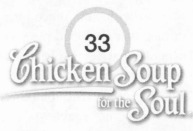

33

A Commitment to Myself

Success means having the courage, the determination, and the will to become the person you believe you were meant to be.

~George Sheehan

Hi, my name is Jeri. I'm a food addict. Not only am I a food addict, I am a food behavior addict. But here's the exciting part. In spite of being a lifelong food behavior addict, I've lost 170 pounds. Picture it—that's 680 sticks of butter kicked to the curb. How did I do it?

Well... I did not have gastric bypass surgery. I did not have lap band surgery. I did not use drugs. I did not use miracle diet gimmicks.

This is how I did it: Diet and Exercise. And water. And therapy and a support group. And journaling, crying. A whole lot of crying in the beginning. In other words, I did it the old fashioned way, the boring way, the my-insurance-won't-pay-for-surgery way. For my food plan, I followed the Jenny Craig plan. My exercise plan consisted of my own two feet walking, and my bike. I was a gym member but cancelled. I figured why pay money to walk on a treadmill and ride an exercise bike when I can do those things for free?

I didn't make a commitment to a program or a plan. I made a commitment to myself. A commitment that no matter what, I was going to do this. I was going to figure out what the heck had been eating at me all these years so I could be done with emotional eating.

My first step was going to my doctor, who sent me to a therapist, who sent me to Jenny Craig. My therapist told me to let her worry about my head and let Jenny worry about my food and, to me, that made sense. My food taken care of, my therapist and I tackled the head game. The game that says if you think you're fat, you are fat and you will behave accordingly. I didn't like that game anymore so I started playing another one. The I-am-so-worth-all-this-fuss game.

I discovered that weight loss is a mental game and willpower has very little to do with it. For me, willpower means white-knuckling my way through life, whereas if I change my thinking with regard to food and put food in its proper place—as merely fuel for my body—I will find lasting success.

I also employed *The Secret* to lose weight, putting into the Universe that I was attracting better health. I told the Universe, "I continue to attract my optimum weight. Whatever weight that is, that's what I'm attracting. The best weight for my body." Then I started envisioning my thin self. I thought up slogans, mantras, and Jeri-isms. Like, "Food is not my friend. Food is not my comforter, nor is it my confidante. It doesn't sing to me or give me wisdom. It's just food. And I am more powerful than food."

I told myself that no matter what life threw at me, I would not gain weight. No matter what! I learned a better way to cope with my emotions. I emote, then get over it. I journal about it, then close the chapter. I move on. And when I sometimes feel a little low, I re-read my journal and re-visit my pictures so I can impress myself all over again. I've learned it's okay to be impressed with myself!

I have learned that when my stomach growls, I will not die. I have learned that there are PEOPLE at parties just five short feet away from the food table to talk to if I just walk away from the table! I have learned that looking good really does taste better than a pound of peanut M&Ms. I have learned that telling myself I am the most beautiful woman on the planet and then behaving accordingly is not a puffed up mind-set, but an empowered one. And who can argue when the results of my head games are staring them in the face?

Now that I have "reached maintenance," I play maintenance

games too. Like, Yes, I can have those chocolate-covered macadamia nuts—but I can only have them in Hawaii. Yes, I can have cake. But I can only eat cake at a wedding, or a birthday party. I can't bake a cake, buy one, or take leftovers home from a party. Yes, I can have one or two pieces of candy brought into the office—but I can't buy candy. Yes, I can have one slice of pizza at a luncheon, but I can't have a pizza delivered to the house. Give and take. Not so rigid, just a little more controlled.

So am I cured? Am I done with all this dieting? I've lost 170 pounds so you'd think I'd be cured. Alas, my food addiction is not cured—but it is managed. I can handle managed.

~Jeri Chrysong

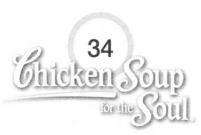

34

Lightening My Load

Could we change our attitude, we should not only see life differently,
but life itself would come to be different.
~Katherine Mansfield

D r. Nath walked into the waiting room to address the family. He looked at the empty fried chicken buckets, cheeseburger wrappers and greasy napkins. Then his gaze shifted from the fast food remnants to the swollen eyes of Claire's family members and he spoke.

"This how she got here, you know. We don't eat like this in India. That is the big difference between us and Americans."

For almost two months, my family, ironically enough, sat in the waiting room and ate as they waited for news about my aunt. Claire had undergone gastric bypass surgery, a last resort in an attempt to lose weight because she was morbidly obese.

But there were complications during and after surgery. Instead of healing and being sent home with post-op directions and a new diet plan, Claire was septic and in the intensive care unit fighting for her life.

Claire's sisters and children took turns sitting with her and holding her hand. And whoever was not with her at the moment was making a run to the nearest fast food restaurant. They ate to maintain a sense of normalcy. They ate as a source of comfort. And they ate to pass the time.

Nearly every female in my family is overweight and I am no exception. I have been fighting my weight since college and I am losing. As soon as I stop paying attention to calories and fat grams, the pounds start creeping up. And before I know it, I have gained 20 pounds.

The signs of weight gain always begin in my face. And that's unfortunate because it is the one place I cannot hide. My cheeks puff out and my chin doubles and soon enough, it's obvious to everyone that I have been eating too much.

The truth is that I love food. I love to eat—a lot. I eat to celebrate. I eat when I am depressed, bored, angry, and upset. Sometimes, it seems as though my stomach knows no limits. I eat salty snacks and sweets. And though I do like the foods that are good for me, I rarely choose them when I have more palate-pleasing options.

Mealtime, for me, is more than obtaining nutrients and sustaining life. I don't eat to live; I live to eat. I often plan my entire day around meals and I get very excited about them.

Just as I have perfected the art of weight gain, I have also gotten very good at shedding extra pounds. Throughout the years, I have tried weight loss pills, meal replacement shakes, and low-carbohydrate diets. I have eaten foods that were low in fat and high in fiber while counting calories, fat grams, and points. I have lost weight. And I have gained it back.

A couple of years ago, I joined a local weight loss group. I thought it would help to be in the presence of other people whose minds operated similarly to mine. I met Mary, the lady who woke up in the middle of the night (every night) to eat a sandwich. I empathized with Jen who stopped at Krispy Kreme after work, bought two dozen doughnuts, then ate one dozen and threw the box away before she arrived home. And then there was Leanne, the woman who often ate two dinners—one in private and a second when she went out with friends. That way, no one would know how much she really consumed. I identified with her most.

Going to group was very successful for me in the beginning. There was something about being held accountable each week (monetarily and to the scale) that kept me motivated. But the key to group settings is that you have to actually go to the meetings. And when I quit going, I started gaining.

A recent trip to the doctor confirmed what I already knew.

"You need to lose about 25 pounds," Dr. Nath said. "You know your family history."

I did know.

Fortunately, my aunt Claire did recover from her surgery. But because the process went so terribly wrong, the gastric bypass was never completed and she has not been able to lose the weight on her own.

My aunt's situation was definitely atypical. Still, I don't want to wait until surgery is my only option to do something about my weight. I also don't want to take the same approaches to weight loss that I have in the past. It is time for a change—a change of body and of mind.

From now on, I am going to think of my body as more than an 18-wheeler on a giant set of scales that either passes or fails inspection. My body is more valuable than that.

Instead, I will eat foods that are rich in vitamins and nutrients. I will drink more water. And, I will exercise by swimming laps at the local pool, taking walks with my husband and dog, and dancing around my living room.

I am not proclaiming that I will never again eat a glazed doughnut. I know I will. But I am gradually making a life change and one that I can live with.

Today I stepped on the scale for the first time since I changed my attitude. I have lost the equivalent of a sack of flour. I know it's just a start; but, it's still worthy of celebration. My body weighs five pounds less. My mind and my heart feel even lighter.

~Melissa Face

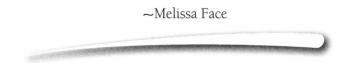

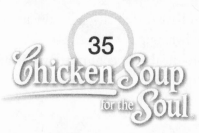

35

Another Loop

*Most people never run far enough on their first wind to find out
they've got a second.*
~William James

My jeans zipper just slid down. I'm not kidding. I am sitting on the couch and my pants just undid themselves. I am on a two-week vacation in Paris and I think a week and a half is all my body can take of carbohydrate wonderland. I add "eat a salad for lunch" to my to-do list. Before my pants rudely interrupted me, I was reading the back of the Nutella jar searching for a 1-800 number. I think I need to admit myself to the Nutella Overeaters Anonymous club. I have demolished eight jars of Nutella in the past 11 days and I have no desire to stop. It is a milk-chocolate hazelnut spread that the French use like peanut butter. I imagine it is supposed to be used sparingly but I don't seem to understand this concept. My body doesn't seem to care either. In fact it is the one that tells me to go buy more. It knows I will sign up for another triathlon, half marathon or century ride, and the weight will balance out. In fact my body is delighted I am treating it to such a reward. Even still, I cannot take it anymore, I did not come to Paris to sit, and so I dig out my running shoes and go for a light jog.

My goal today is 20 minutes. Any workout is better than none, right? If I can at least keep this going for approximately two miles then I can call it a day. As I am huffing down the street I try not to concentrate on the torture I am inflecting on myself. I realize that running is by far the best metaphor for life. Sometimes it is fun, effortless and rewarding; other times it is pure abuse and agony. Today my calves feel like lead. I think all the chocolate and cheese has molded together and formed a hard rock in my body. As torturous as this is, I know I must keep pushing through. I am approaching the 20-minute mark, and I tell myself to go around one more time. I relocated to Montmartre a few days ago. So my new running path is around the outside of the Montmartre Cemetery. Once around the outside, which is what I call the loop, is a little more than a mile. It takes me about 10 minutes to run all the way around. So I tell myself to go around one more time and then I can quit.

As I turn the corner, there is a young man who looks up and smiles at me. He sprints to catch up and jogs along with me for a few moments. He has a giant goofy grin, which in return produces a silly grin on my face. He says a few words in French. I just point to my earphones to show I am listening to music, so that I won't have to reveal that I don't speak French. I am enchanted with this young man. He is running along with a perfect stranger just for the fun of it. I decide to make him my running angel. He is here to entertain me and keep me smiling as I push myself on this run.

I look down at my watch and realize I have been running for 55 minutes. For the past half hour I have been so engrossed in the moment that I actually forgot I was running. I have taken a measly 20-minute run and turned it into a strong 60-minute workout.

~Shannon Kaiser

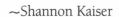

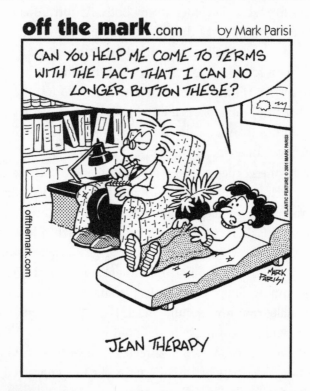

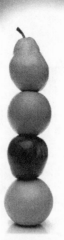

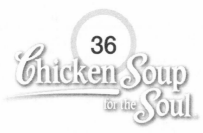

No Excuses

The human body is the only machine
for which there are no spare parts.
~Hermann M. Biggs

I got into the exercise habit as a twenty-year-old college student, and it has stayed with me nearly 40 years. My sense of identity was very much tied up in that healthy image, and if anyone had asked me along the way, I'd have said I was a runner—or later on, a walker. Oddly enough, that self-image remained even when daily reality became something else altogether.

Oh, I still walked. But walks that used to be miles now were often just a half-mile... or even less. Life just got too busy—I was working as an attorney, and had a long commute. I traveled a lot for my job and it was hard to figure out where to squeeze in a work-out, between flying across the country, breakfast meetings, and long evenings of strategizing. I remember trying to run in place in my hotel room while my colleagues were at the bar before dinner, but it wasn't enough. Other times, I got up early and did loops around the hotel. Even when I was home, it was often dark and I was tired, so a quarter-mile turn between our house and the neighbors' was the extent of my daily exercise.

The arrival of my three babies within a two-year period was even more devastating. I struggled to survive on as little as four hours sleep a night, and before I knew it, I was back commuting to work again.

What I found was that life intervened. If it wasn't work, it was kids. If it wasn't kids, it was two weeks of flu—or a death in the family. Or any number of other things. There was always a reason—or an excuse—for abbreviating my workout or just skipping it. Every time, I told myself that as soon as the present crisis was over, I would get back into my routine. Meanwhile, I was a healthy person, I told myself. After all, I worked out!

Amazingly, I was able to keep telling myself this—and believing it—even after "the present crisis" stretched into a matter of years. My asthma, which had plagued me in my 20s and then seemed to vanish, came back with a vengeance after a bad bout with a virus. My hips and lower back ached night and day, to the point where I had to struggle to get out of bed, or even to tie my shoes. Between my joint pain and my breathing issues, I had trouble sleeping.

One day, I woke up and looked around me. I was horrified to realize I felt old. Of course, at this point, 20 years of "temporary" distractions had come between me and any serious attempt to exercise. I was still eating the way I always had, but suddenly, my weight was creeping up, and I'd developed the most distressing potbelly—it was actually so pronounced that I could have set my plate on it and eaten standing up. Now when I couldn't sleep at night, I used the time to worry about whether I was already starting the dying process.

Determined, I started increasing my daily walks. Instead of the quick quarter-mile, I did a full mile most days—or even a mile and a half from time to time. But to my consternation, I didn't feel much better. I saw the doctor for my asthma and my chiropractor for my joints. And I bumped up my exercise again. I walked faster, trying to do my mile in under 15 minutes. After I got used to that, I stretched my walk to two miles, then three. By the end of summer, I was doing my three miles in under 45 minutes.

I was amazed at how quickly I started feeling better, and how fast my potbelly shrank to a less scary size. My old sense of myself as strong, healthy, and energetic had returned!

But walking that far and that fast was work. I had to push myself when I was tired, when it was hot and muggy—or dank and rainy. I really wasn't enjoying my workouts a lot of the time, and I wondered how long I'd be able to keep pushing myself through them.

Then, one day, I learned my high school friend had died of breast cancer. She'd been two years younger than me, and she was gone. I'd had the flu again, and afterward, my lungs just never really cleared. Months went by, and I felt as if I was drowning in heavy mucus. Maybe it was because I was thinking about my friend, but as an ex-smoker I became convinced I had lung cancer. After all, my father had had both lung cancer and emphysema when he'd died—and my mother's sister, who had never been a smoker, had had lung cancer, as well.

Because I'd had this deep cough for so long, my doctor ordered a CT scan. Instead of reassuring me, it revealed multiple areas of density. My doctor's voice showed how concerned she was—I'd need a bronchoscopy.

Fleeing my demons, I walked longer, harder, faster. I walked in all kinds of weather, concentrating on deep breaths as I ferociously charged ahead, my face pouring sweat or stung by raindrops, or with snow piling up inside my glasses. I would outwalk this; I would.

After my bronchoscopy, and another year of CT scans, I was released with a diagnosis of benign nodules, and I felt reborn. I kept walking my fast and furious miles—until we went on a long vacation… and then, I got sick again. And then, my mother went into the hospital and I had to drive back and forth for many weeks. Life, once again, had intervened.

I kept trying to get a consistent routine going, but every time I did, the next crisis hit. Besides, I really didn't enjoy working that hard.

At this point, another friend gave me the push I needed. Because of a chronic lung condition, she was on oxygen, and needed a wheelchair in order to handle long distances. She asked me to accompany her on a round of appointments at Cleveland Clinic. From early morning until six at night, I pushed her from one test to another, one appointment to another. By the end of the day, I was sitting waiting for her last consultation. As I sat there, I watched all the patients, both young and old, as they came and went in their wheelchairs or leaning on walkers or companions, trailing oxygen tanks or wearing paper masks against infection.

Suddenly, I was struck right in the very pit of my stomach by how fortunate I am—and shame washed over me. There I'd been, so quick to let my exercise routine get derailed by inconvenience, so quick to whine and complain about how hard it was. What person in that waiting room wouldn't have cried with joy and relief to be able to do what I do—the way I myself had felt when I got that benign diagnosis? And who wouldn't want to work hard, the way I once had, to be able to stay that way?

Since that day, all I need do to get myself back on track is to put myself back in that waiting room. With each sweaty, straining step, I say, "Thank you, Lord!" and push on.

~Susan Kimmel Wright

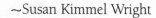

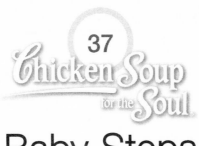

Baby Steps

Motherhood has a very humanizing effect.
Everything gets reduced to essentials.
~Meryl Streep

I was in the habit of taking pregnancy tests. For two years my husband and I tried to have a baby with no success. We kept our cupboard stocked with the home kits and every month I would give a cursory glance at the negative sign and throw it in the trash. I repeated this familiar routine one day in the fall of 2005 when, to my surprise, my test was positive.

I went into the living room where my husband Jimmy was watching TV, sat down beside him and stared at that positive sign as it shook in my jittery hands. Jimmy let out a whoop when he saw the test, and then he became quiet too. I don't know how long we both sat there, gazing at our unexpected gift.

The day I went to my obstetrician to confirm my pregnancy was balmy and fresh, a sign, I thought, of the happiness to come. I arrived more than 30 minutes early and had to wait a long time to see the doctor. She came into my examination room with her face buried in my paperwork.

"You're pregnant, Mrs. Reese."

I grinned and waited for the congratulations I knew were coming next. Instead, my doctor frowned at me.

"It's dangerous to become pregnant at your weight. You need to be very careful if you want to have a healthy pregnancy."

She continued with a daunting recitation of the hazards of being overweight and pregnant. She talked about miscarriages and birth defects, all the while writing down an overwhelming list of rules for me to follow.

Twenty-five minutes later, my doctor handed me the list and looked up from her sheaf of papers. She seemed suddenly aware that I hadn't spoken since our visit began.

"Are you all right, Nancy?"

It took all of my strength to nod my head and keep my tears at bay. The doctor moved to leave the room, and as she brushed past me, she squeezed my arm.

"Congratulations."

I barely made it to my car before erupting into tears. My girl-friends who had babies before me were elated after their first doctor's visits. Many of them celebrated their pregnancies by picking out baby names or nursery colors.

I began my pregnancy feeling like I had already failed my baby.

As I sobbed in my car, I was confronted with all the years of pain and hopelessness I had suffered due to my weight problems. Overweight since I was seven years old, I had countless memories of feeling broken because I was fat. From being the last one picked in gym class to being overlooked for job opportunities, my past was cluttered with images of people measuring me by my weight and finding me inadequate. Still, none of those experiences prepared me for the thought of beginning motherhood as a bad mom.

When I ran out of tears, I began my drive home. I tried to be rational and evaluate my situation, but my sorrow was so intense that I felt paralyzed. Suddenly, right before I arrived at home, an epiphany pierced through my sadness. I realized I was acting like a victim and that I had been a victim for a very long time. I realized it wasn't really my weight that held me back all those years, but my own inability to empower myself enough to change. Most importantly, I realized that if I didn't make serious and immediate changes in my life, my baby would be a victim too.

I became a survivor that day.

During my pregnancy, I took better care of myself than I ever had before. Every meal was an opportunity to nourish my baby and every movement was a chance to strengthen my body. My obstetrician was thrilled with my progress — my blood pressure stayed consistently low and my weight gain was on target. I was doing so well, in fact, that after my first trimester, my doctor decided my pregnancy was no longer considered high risk.

In the spring of 2006, my son Ben was born. He was healthy, beautiful and happy right from the start. I was fortunate to spend the first three months of Ben's life at home with him, doing all the "usual" things that make those early days so extraordinary. Every sound he uttered convinced me he was a genius; every bath resulted in a photo shoot; every smile was a miracle.

I had returned to my pre-pregnancy weight by the time my maternity leave was over, and was faced with yet another revelation: My health was still at risk, and now my life was about more than just me.

I wanted the stamina to keep up with Ben when he grew into an energetic toddler, to live to see him mature into a man. I also wanted to set a great example of health and fitness for my son.

Before I was pregnant, I tried every fad diet out there and failed at permanent weight loss every time. So, for six months I researched weight loss and exercise methods and carved a path I thought would work for me. I knew I needed a solid plan that was tailored for my personality if I was going to succeed. Finally, I was able to put my strategy into action.

It's not easy to make up for a lifetime of poor eating habits and sedentary behavior. I had a lot of success when I began this journey and the pounds were coming off quickly and steadily. But as I get closer to my goal and the weight loss slows, it's been a challenge not to go back to my old ways. Fortunately, I have a very good reason not to give up on myself: a bouncy, curly-haired three-year-old.

Today, I am 60 pounds lighter than I was before I got pregnant. Losing another 30 pounds is still a part of my plan, and it can be quite daunting to consider how much further I have to go. I try not to dwell on the long road ahead; instead I simply try to make one healthy decision at a time.

Ben and I were putting some of his baby clothes into storage recently, and we came across a stack of old photos. He picked up a pre-pregnancy picture of me, and asked, "Mommy, who's that?" When I told him it was me, he shook his head and answered with the kind of blind confidence only three-year-olds possess. "That's not my mommy!" I wrapped my arms around my son and said a prayer of thanks that Ben's mommy is, indeed, very different from the woman in the picture. I am so grateful to have improved my health and quality of life, and I'm blessed to have a little boy who inspires me to live fearlessly.

~Nancy Higgins Reese

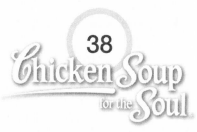

Instant Willpower

A deadline is negative inspiration.
Still, it's better than no inspiration at all.
~Rita Mae Brown

"T his is for you," Al said. My husband handed me a thick envelope. I lifted the flap and discovered two tickets inside for a Western Caribbean seven-day cruise.

"Happy 30th anniversary," Al said.

"Wow! Thank you." I kissed him. "But, isn't our anniversary six months away?"

"Well, the travel agent said you have to reserve these trips far in advance."

We had cruised two years earlier, and visions of midnight buffet tables made my stomach rumble. I had gained 10 pounds in five days and never lost them.

The following weekend, when we were babysitting my four-year-old granddaughter she asked, "Grandma, why are you fat?" I gasped.

"Grandma likes her goodies," I replied and faked a smile.

Monday morning, I examined my body in front of the full-length mirror. Oh, no. When did that potbelly arrive? Checking the side view, I saw fat jiggle on my butt, thighs, and arms. Parts of me sagged. I studied my plump face; a double chin reflected back at me. Stepping on my scale, I watched the number rise higher than ever before. My scale refused to lie. I'd gained a total of 45 pounds. My self-image took a nosedive.

The mirror told the truth. At fifty-eight, I had ballooned out of shape. No wonder most of my clothes didn't fit. Menopause had seized my body and layered it in fat.

One afternoon I saw a magazine cover at the grocery store: "Instant Willpower. Are you always hungry but can't lose weight?" Yes, I whispered. Beneath the eye-catching statement, a pretty, thin brunette stood next to her "before" picture. She touted a 50-pound weight loss. Skeptical, I purchased the issue anyway.

At bedtime, I read and reread the article. The thin woman based her willpower theory on a meditation plan. Many years ago, I had meditated for stress and it worked for me. I devoured her dieting tricks, but still had my doubts. My looming anniversary cruise forced me to make a decision. Could I summon up the strength to shed the weight? I drifted off to sleep thinking positive, reaffirming thoughts.

The next day, I retrieved a brand new four-subject notebook from my desk. I labeled the first tab as my food journal. The second, I dedicated to fitness workouts, the third for logging weekly weight loss. In the last section I scribbled my reasons for obtaining this goal and then listed my reward. As a deterrent, I cut out the thin model and the words "Instant Willpower" and stuck them on my refrigerator.

Motivated, I meditated for 15 minutes and repeated my mantra, Instant Willpower. Each time I had a food craving, I shoved a piece of sugar-free gum into my mouth. My love affair with carbohydrates had made me an addict. The first couple of weeks were tough.

The article also recommended getting fit and suggested personal trainers, but I couldn't afford one. So I searched the Internet for examples of training plans. A free trainer website offered a regular exercise regime and the number of calories burned. I grabbed my notebook and entered a column for each: walking, jogging, bike riding and swimming. I couldn't remember the last time I did any physical activity.

I shopped at thrift stores and purchased a used bicycle, a jump rope and a pedometer. Before dinner, I walked two miles at a regular pace. An aroma coming from a neighbor's barbecue conjured up a mental image of hamburgers, potato salad and baked beans. I could almost taste the meal. I grabbed a stick of mint gum and chewed away the craving. I pictured myself sunning on a deck chair, alongside my husband, wearing a new bathing suit. It worked.

After the first month, I walked in the mornings. I mixed walking a block and jogging the next and gradually increased my distance to four miles. The temperature was cooler and the odors different. I inhaled the scent of fresh-cut grass. Alone with my thoughts, I meditated, repeating my mantra over and over in my mind. The hunger pains disappeared. I biked an hour each evening and the ride invigorated me. Instead of considering exercise a chore, I incorporated the activity into my new lifestyle. Four months later, the scale showed a 30-pound weight loss. I entered the number in my log, a wide grin on my face. Only 15 more pounds to reach my goal.

I stuck to the magazine's rigid diet and recipes, although at times I found myself standing and staring at the fridge. I'd recite my mantra and study the thin smiling model. I reaffirmed my goal by writing my feelings in my notebook and then brushed my teeth. A well-known diet trick, but it kept me from cheating.

One night my husband said, "You're looking good." The compliment made me blush. I continued eating fruits, veggies, chicken and grains, but nothing white. Carbohydrates were the enemy. At night, I swore off television and enjoyed catching up on my reading pile. I heard the less food you see, the less hungry you are. It worked for me.

As the pounds dropped off, I had more energy. In the afternoon, I swam laps at our clubhouse pool or jumped rope in my backyard. For the first time in years, I experienced the childhood thrill of simple pleasures. Five months and three weeks passed. I had lost 45 pounds and met my goal. As promised, I splurged and shopped for a new wardrobe for our cruise.

Our anniversary arrived and together we boarded the ship. A cameraman stopped us for a boarding photograph. My husband beamed and slipped his arm around my thin waist. Once we settled inside our cabin, he smiled and said, "Wow, you look even better than the day we got married. Happy 30th anniversary; think of this as our second honeymoon." We hugged and kissed.

My heart pounded faster. I remembered doubting that magazine headline, Instant Willpower, now my mantra forever. I opened my suitcase holding the new size-6 cruise wear. The first thing I unpacked was my four-subject notebook.

~Suzanne Baginskie

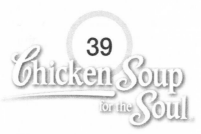

39

Resolution Not Revolution

Small deeds done are better than great deeds planned.
~Peter Marshall

Eight, 10, 12, 14... year after year, I watched my jean size creep up, along with the number on the bathroom scale. Feeling weak and ashamed, I responded by exercising like gangbusters and severely limiting my caloric intake. I would promptly lose five to 10 pounds, and then slowly fall back into my old habits—overeating and infrequent exercising. Falling back into bad habits meant falling back into larger jeans, too.

In late 2006, I began to think about my previous attempts at weight loss. I realized my goals were always too demanding and I was inadvertently setting myself up to fail. In previous years, I had told myself that I would lose 10 pounds by the end of January, five more pounds by the end of February, five more by the end of March and so on. I set a much different kind of goal for January 2007.

I vowed to walk on the treadmill for 15 minutes at least five days a week. It was a small, manageable goal. I began walking just two miles per hour for 15 minutes, giving myself the weekends off. I worked my way up to three miles per hour for 15 minutes and then three miles per hour for 20 minutes. Month after month, little by little, I increased my rate of speed and the length of my walk. I now walk four miles per hour for 30 minutes each day.

I added another manageable goal for January 2008. I had been drinking at least one soda every day. I wanted to drink less soda and more water. Again, I cut back little by little, month after month, and over the course of the year, I reduced my consumption to just one soda a week.

In January 2009 I set myself another new fitness goal. Previously, I was eating fast food two to three times each week. I knew that if I could manage to scale that back, I would be doing my body and my pocketbook a huge favor. Again, just like with my previous goals, I cut back little by little. After two months, I was already down to eating out just once a week.

After just two years on my journey to a new and healthier lifestyle, I was down 20 pounds and comfortably back into my size 8 jeans. By keeping my goals small, I was able to follow through and sustain each one for the long haul. I continue to see the results on the scale, and I feel so much better with each passing year and each new resolution!

~Kimberly M. Hutmacher

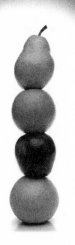

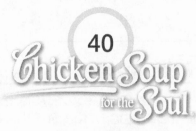

40

Twenty Pounds and Counting

You can't lose weight by talking about it. You have to keep your mouth shut.
~Author Unknown

C alories have always loved me. In fact, they worshipped me, using my body as their temple and congregating around my waist, hips, and thighs. The more they adored me, the more I expanded.

In those days, my mantra was: "Calories? Who knows? Who cares?" The more junk food I ate, the louder I chanted. And with each pound representing 3,500 calories, and my being 20 pounds overweight, I was doing a lot of chanting and chewing to have picked up 70,000 freeloaders, er, acolytes.

Nice as it is to be loved, even adoration has its drawbacks. I had to buy new jeans with an extra relaxed fit to accommodate me and my gang of acolytes.

Not wanting to be a card-carrying member of Generation O for obesity, and worried that my freeloaders would invite friends to join them at the altar of my hips, I put down the remote control and joined a gym. Decked out in sweatpants and oversized T-shirt, I prepared to pare down.

The gang and I pedaled for miles on the stationary bike; we climbed uphill and downhill on the treadmill; and we lifted weights until our muscles screamed in protest. Rather MY muscles screamed;

the fat cells just bunched over my waistband and hung on for dear life.

The gang wasn't thrilled about this new routine. About 17,500 of them packed their bags and left, presumably to find someone who didn't shake them up, down, and sideways. But the other 52,500 stayed. Either they were made of sterner stuff or they assumed I would get tired of working out and head back for the couch.

I didn't.

For the next three years, I averaged two and a third trips to the gym per week. The mirror told me I looked better, and I traded a relaxed pant for one that didn't shout "overweight." But I couldn't shake my most devoted acolytes.

I ignored the fact that I rewarded myself with junk food after a workout. Sometimes I rewarded myself with junk food for merely thinking about going to the gym. After eating a family-sized bag of chips, your body doesn't want to lift anything heavier than the empty package.

When I stepped on the scale, I told myself the "weight" was muscle. After all, a pec flex produced a lump that was at least the size of a lemon. Almost.

Then my gym offered a 10-week nutrition/weight loss course. I signed up. The come-on: "10 pounds in 10 weeks," was enticing. I figured if I paid $200 for the course, I might actually follow the advice and evict another 35,000 unwanted acolytes.

At the first session, the instructor handed out weekly food-tracking sheets and I realized my days of ignoring food labels were over. I'd have to weigh and measure every mouthful, track the ratio of protein, carbs, and fat, and write it all down. Worse, someone else would know everything I put in my mouth.

If that weren't bad enough, I'd be weighed every session — on a scale that could tell fat from muscle. I almost asked for my money back, but the tightness in my waistband persuaded me to go ahead with the course. That and the gym's no-money-back policy.

The next morning, I placed food lists on my fridge door, got out my measuring cups and spoons, and girded my loins for war: Harriet against her temple acolytes.

At the grocery store, I read the nutrition labels on every item before allowing it in my shopping cart and finally learned how much fat and carbs were packed into a single bag of chips. Not wanting to live at the gym for the rest of my life, I bade goodbye to the chips, and headed for the fresh produce section.

I also chanted my new mantra: "Twenty grams protein, 30 grams carbs, and 10 grams fat" at every meal until I thought my head would explode. I cubed low-fat cheese into strict one-serving portions. I ate raw veggies until my jaws ached from the constant crunching. I ditched the deep fryer and grilled chicken, shrimp, and tofu burgers.

After 10 weeks, I'd lost eight pounds and I kept on losing. By the time I'd lost 15 pounds, I had memorized the food charts and no longer needed to record every mouthful. After 20 pounds, I had to buy new clothes.

While it's gotten easier, it's never gotten easy. I keep a picture of myself taken 20 years ago next to my computer. The woman in the picture is slim, not skinny, and she's smiling. That's the woman I want to be, not the woman who spent years hiding from cameras because she didn't like what she saw.

Luckily, I've developed a taste for raw veggies, low-fat cheese, and grilled chicken. And if the odd chip or piece of chocolate crosses my lips, it's not the end of world. I warn any would-be acolytes that they're short-term and not to unpack their bags.

The next day I chant my mantra a little louder.

~Harriet Cooper

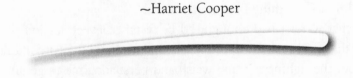

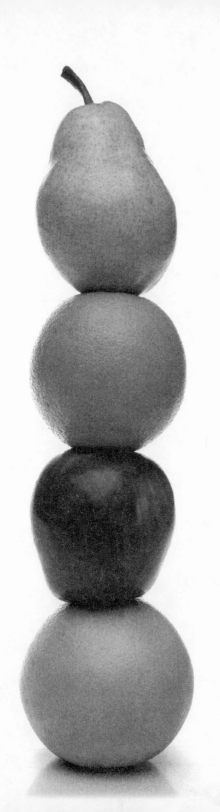

Shaping the New You

The Gym

*I have 24 hours in each of my days
just like everyone else.
It's how I choose to use those hours
that will make the difference in my days.*

~*Richard Simmons*, The Book of Hope

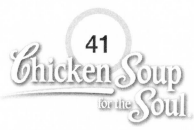

41

Conquering the Gym

Too many people confine their exercise to jumping to conclusions,
running up bills, stretching the truth, bending over backward, lying down on
the job, sidestepping responsibility and pushing their luck.

~Anonymous

A fat girl in elementary school is lined up against a painted cinderblock wall with her classmates. Two boys—the best athletes in the class, of course—stand several feet away, surveying the group critically. One by one, the students are called to join the boys' teams, until only one student is left. "Nancy," one of the boys mumbles. The girl keeps her eyes on the ground, too embarrassed to look at anyone, as she joins her team.

These are the images that pop into my head, so many years later, when I think of myself in a gym. Anyone who's been a fat kid knows gym is the worst place to be. So, last year when my diet buddy suggested that we join the gym that's housed in our office building, I literally laughed in her face. "No way!" I said, without even thinking about it. When she asked for an explanation I told her it would devastate my weight loss efforts. "Kimmy, the moment I go in there and get laughed at, I will feel like a failure. I can't take that kind of pressure right now. I need to keep things positive."

I was working so hard on my journey to reach a healthy weight. I had already lost 60 pounds, but I had at least another 30 to go before I would be satisfied. I felt that any negativity could derail me entirely, and my experience with gyms had never been anything but negative.

She let it go, and I thought—hoped—that would be the end of it. But my diet buddy is nothing if not persistent. Every month or two she would find a new tactic to try to convince me to go to the gym. At first she touted how inexpensive our gym is, and that I'd never find a better deal anywhere else.

"I don't want to find a better deal," I snapped. "I'm never going to the gym."

Then she tried to convince me that it wasn't that kind of gym. "There are people of all sizes and skill levels at this gym, Nancy. Everybody does their own thing, and nobody pays attention to anyone else." But how could a girl like me believe that? I knew that as soon as I walked through the door, the big, athletic guys and the tiny, perfect girls would instantly see who I was: a fat fourth-grader whose only goal at the gym was to be as invisible as possible until I could leave.

One day, during the holiday season, I was foolish enough to complain about how little time I had to work out. I tried to do it when I got my son to bed at night, but by that time I'm usually wiped out. And I'd just had an extremely unsuccessful two weeks of attempting to work out at 5 a.m. before my family woke up. But since I am nearly unable to function before 8 a.m., I was a zombie during my workouts and was quite literally going through the motions, with almost no benefit to my body.

"You know, there's a really easy solution to your problem," Kimmy replied. Her latest strategy was to proclaim the convenience of being able to work out during our lunch hour. As I came up with one excuse after another from my impressive arsenal, she sat silently and listened to all the words she'd heard before. She was very quiet when she said, "Nancy, it doesn't have to be this complicated. You're not a kid anymore, and this doesn't have to own you."

And in that moment, I knew she was right. As much progress as I'd made, I knew I would never be able to reach my goal weight, let alone keep it off, without conquering all the old demons that still haunted me. I needed to step out of my comfort zone. I realized it was my comfort zone, and not some elementary school bullies, that kept me from succeeding.

Four weeks ago I started at the gym, and I have to be honest with you: I was absolutely terrified. When Kimmy and I arrived, it was already crowded. People were lifting weights, running on the treadmills, and cycling imaginary miles on the stationary bikes. A man on the elliptical machine was shouting to his friend about how hard it is to do "two 18s" in a row. A woman jumped off the treadmill with her first two fingers poked into her neck. And I started to panic. What if somebody wants to talk to me about "two 18s?" I don't even know what that is! Should I poke my neck too? Am I checking to see if it's still fat?

Kimmy and I put our DVD into the player and started to warm up. It was surprisingly fun to work out with a buddy, much more entertaining than doing the DVD by myself. Between the music from our DVD, the sounds of all the machines and people talking, it got pretty loud at the gym and the scary thoughts in my mind began to fade.

Four weeks later, I don't hear those thoughts much anymore. The big guys that were so intimidating on my first day give me a warm wave when I arrive now; and the super-skinny girl that rules the elliptical machine confessed that she's never been confident enough to use workout DVDs in front of everybody. I told her she can join us any time. Fourth grade was a long time ago for everybody I see at the gym. As far as I can tell, no one is thinking about dividing into teams or deciding who is the weakest link. At this stage, everyone is really there to work on their own goals—health, weight loss, empowerment and strength.

And although I will always remember the little girl who was picked last, I can now look at myself in the floor-to-ceiling mirrors at the gym and see just how far I've come.

~Nancy Higgins Reese

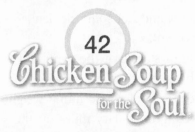

42

Saddle Sore

Endurance is not just the ability to bear a hard thing,
but to turn it into glory.
~William Barclay

The jolly winter holidays led me to ply myself with much comforting food and drink. While I indulged in this munch-a-rama, my entire wardrobe shrank—in some cases, by a whole size. At first, I thought I might have just left the clothes in the dryer for too long. But then someone left the bathroom scale in a place I was sure to see it: in front of the refrigerator. Not the most tactful hint in the world, but unmistakable in its meaning.

After wasting an hour on deep relaxation exercises, I stepped on the scale and discovered that sucking in the gut while being weighed does nothing to reduce the fateful number. Whoever claimed that broken chocolate chip cookies didn't have as many calories as whole cookies was wrong—tragically wrong.

The worst punishment I could imagine was going to a spinning class. The fitness industry doesn't want this to get around, but when torture chambers have been discovered in various nefarious places, alongside the cattle prods and other painful devices, they have found two dozen recumbent bicycles and a whole slew of CDs filled with the techno-rap "music" they play in spinning classes. Heck, anybody would confess to the most heinous crimes imaginable after listening to that stuff long enough. Given the problem of prison overcrowding, why not sentence our most hardened criminals to 15 years in the nearest fitness center, where the only activity would be spinning classes? No college education, no making license plates, no new tattoos, just spinning, all day, every day. I bet you the entire federal deficit that those ne'er-do-wells would finally understand what it means to get tough on crime.

To say that I hate spinning is a huge understatement, but how could I argue with the opportunity to burn a whopping 400 calories in one hour? I hauled my bigger self to the gym and straddled the only bike left unoccupied in the class. Fortunately, this bike was in the back of the room, so that few people would notice, and perhaps pity, the unsightly panty lines showing through my Spandex pants.

The instructor was already shouting instructions: "Give me 30 seconds in a 2 o'clock position!" "Now raise the resistance and give me 60 seconds in a 4 o'clock position!" I didn't quite understand the subtle differences between where our fannies were supposed to be at 2 o'clock versus 4 o'clock. Mine would have much preferred to have been on the couch while I savored an Edith Wharton novel. But this was my penalty to pay, so I kept fiddling with the resistance lever, hovering between full aerobic capacity and cardiac arrest.

Melissa, the instructor, yelled, "Are you all feeling GREAT?" It was a rhetorical question, not allowing for any response, and the class was well trained. They whooped and hollered in response, raising their eco-friendly water bottles for a collective, self-congratulatory swig. Melissa drank from a jug big enough to have filled my minivan's gas tank for a week. Frankly, I suspect the spinners just made those whooping noises because no one was capable of forming actual words.

After 10 minutes, I realized that if the workout didn't kill me, the boredom surely would, so I tried a friendly banter with the woman on the bike next to me. Already blessed with a great figure, she was spinning her little thighs into oblivion. "Do you really like this?" I asked, lowering the resistance lever yet again.

"In a kind of masochistic way, I suppose," she laughed. "Hey, does your back hurt?"

"No. Am I doing something wrong?" I began to worry.

"Maybe. It ought to hurt by tomorrow," she promised.

The seconds trudged forward in agonizing slowness. At one point I thought I heard Melissa order us to "move our ovaries" but I was too embarrassed to ask my neighbor if that was what she really said. Anyway, even if she had issued that command, I couldn't exactly expect mine to oblige just on her say-so.

Although I was not as fast as my spinning comrades, I outlasted the weaklings who pooped out, some as much as 15 minutes early. Of course, if they had paced themselves more carefully and not over-exerted, they could have kept on pedaling as long as I did.

As the class eventually spun itself to a merciful conclusion, Melissa offered this helpful safety reminder: "Please do not dismount until your bikes have come to a complete stop. Remember that many body parts may have shifted during class, so be extremely careful during your dismount. We thank you for spinning with Buff Bodies, Inc. and hope that you will spin with us again soon."

At home, I walked in the door like a character in a spaghetti Western, only without the ten-gallon hat. Of course, I must now purge the word "spaghetti" from my vocabulary, except as an adjective describing a kind of shoulder strap that I am unsuited to wear, or the aforementioned type of movie genre.

Today I am walking even funnier than I did yesterday, and many body parts are beginning to ache. The good news is that there is no piece of cake yet invented that could possibly be worth eating if the price is returning to spinning class.

Except, perhaps, for a slice of double chocolate cheesecake.

~Judy Gruen

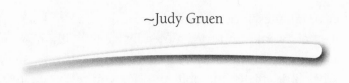

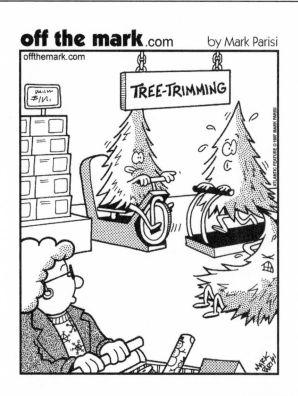

off the mark.com by Mark Parisi

offthemark.com

TREE-TRIMMING

Reprinted by permission of Off the Mark
and Mark Parisi ©1997

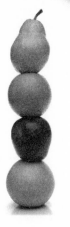

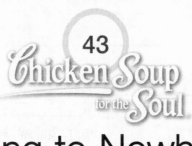

43

Biking to Nowhere

With the heaps of overly specialized gear—
gloves, shoes, and biking jerseys—most cyclists realize that
every day on the road is Halloween.
~Joe Kurmaskie

I recently bought a pair of biking shoes. Not a big deal, you might say. Except I don't own a bike. Instead, twice a week, I engage in an indoor activity called group cycling.

Group cycling, or spinning, is a relatively new exercise regimen built around a specially designed, heavy-duty stationary bicycle. A dozen or more of these bikes are arranged facing a bike-mounted instructor who leads the class participants on an hour-long journey to nowhere.

I figured to be the last person participating in this trendy aerobic exercise. As a fifty-three-year-old, overweight male, I was not looking to be a cutting edge trendsetter. In fact, for many years, my exercise routine centered around such traditional activities as racquetball, squash and exercise classes.

But thanks to all that high-impact exercise, my hips eventually began to wear out. Due to incipient osteoarthritis, I reluctantly gave up racquet sports and switched to something called step aerobics.

It wasn't an easy switch. After all, these were classes populated almost exclusively by women. And they were hard. Learning to master a dozen different tricky moves on an elevated step wasn't the best way to feed my aging masculine ego.

But I persevered and I'm glad I did. Step aerobics is a low-impact exercise routine that provides a great workout. And after a while, I had mastered most of the fancy moves and was "stepping" three times a week.

As with most things, however, I eventually became a bit bored with step classes. Although it still provided a good workout, it was hard to work up enthusiasm for three classes a week. Plus, my aging hips were starting to feel the wear and tear of even this low-impact exercise.

So two years ago I tried my hand at spinning. Without a clue, and lacking proper equipment, I managed to survive my first class although just barely. My lungs were burning, my legs were aching and my butt was sore.

Despite the pain of that first class, I recognized that this might be a good exercise routine to supplement my step classes. For one thing, it didn't stress my hips. And for another, it gave me a great aerobic workout.

So I signed up for one class a week. I solved the burning lungs problem by moderating my pace. The aching legs disappeared once I learned to do extra stretching after the class. And the sore butt was eased with a $20 gel seat.

Before I knew it, I was taking two spinning classes a week and I had cut back my step participation to only once a week. But that was only the beginning.

One of the keys to efficient spinning is to maintain one's heart rate in the preferred aerobic zone. And the preferred method of maintaining a specific heart rate is to use a heart rate monitor. After a year of spinning classes, I was finally convinced to cough up eighty bucks for one of these wristwatch and chest band devices.

At that point I was beginning to feel a bit self-conscious. For someone who doesn't even own a bike, I had now invested $100 in biking equipment.

But that wasn't the end. After another year of stationary travel, different instructors convinced me to spend $120 on bike shoes and clips to achieve more efficient pedaling in my journey without destination.

Despite looking somewhat foolish with all my cycling gear, the instructors' advice proved to be correct. I was now spinning more efficiently and getting a better workout.

As I continue on my indoor cycling travels, I've also realized some non-aerobic benefits. Once you learn how to spin correctly and monitor your heart rate properly, you can sometimes experience an almost meditative state.

When I occasionally achieve what some instructors call the mind-body connection, I close my eyes and find myself drifting away from the everyday worries of life. And on those days when everything seems to click, I can get lost in this other world for minutes at a time.

Once you get the hang of spinning, it provides a double return for your efforts. Not only do you get a great aerobic workout, you also get a stress-relieving break from the outside world and a refreshed psyche ready to tackle life's trials with renewed energy.

More recently, I've even been adding the occasional third weekly spinning class to my regimen. It's an hour and a half endurance ride designed to build my aerobic capacity without pushing me over the cardiac edge.

The problem is that the more I get into group cycling, the more I seem to spend and the sillier I look. Despite a lifelong aversion to Spandex, I'm now realizing that my next purchase will likely be a pair of biking shorts to provide additional comfort to my sometimes aching backside. And then there are the special breathable biking socks and the biking gloves and the fancy water bottle.

No matter how hard I resist, I suspect I'm destined to become a Spandex-clad, bike-shoe-wearing indoor cyclist with all the bells and whistles. And given the benefits I get from spinning my wheels, I guess the embarrassment is ultimately worth it.

Who knows? If I find that I can't take the mortification anymore, I may even have to buy a bike.

~David Martin

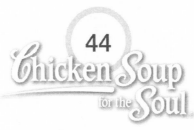

44

I Just Stepped Off

You will never find time for anything. If you want time, you must make it.

~Charles Buxton

"Mommies have a lot of water," my four-year-old announced, wobbling the ample excess of my thighs back and forth.

Sighing, I let the observation stand. I had told him that the human body is composed largely of water, so how could I correct him? Besides, I don't like to call my excess by its proper name. I just don't use F-words.

I attribute many of my rolls and dimples to this adorable child of mine who hasn't got an ounce of fat on him. But although childbirth helped land me in this fix, I must be honest and credit motherhood with getting me out of it. Motherhood changed my idea of time, and with it, my idea of how to reach a goal.

Before Evan was born, I was a typically productive member of the workforce. I was a journalist and a pretty good one, chiefly because I could meet a deadline. You want a story by 5 o'clock? No problem. A few calls, an interview, some pounding of the keys and it's done. The rhythm of my writing days was intense, a non-stop workathon ending at a daily finish line.

Without my even knowing it, this method of goal-setting had infused my entire life. Periodically, I'd resolve to lose a few pounds. I'd start off great, starve myself for hours, but by the end of the day I'd look in the mirror and realize that—surprise!—I hadn't taken off

20 pounds. Hadn't met my unacknowledged and utterly ridiculous deadline. In a huff, I'd stuff myself.

Not surprisingly, I found that the rhythm of a mother's day is not one smooth upward trajectory ending in triumph. Rather, a mother's day is an assemblage of broken hours punctuated by frantic spurts of activity. You dash off a few e-mails during naptime. Make phone calls while Elmo entertains. Planning your day is a relic of the past and nothing you can aspire to in the near future. Inwardly, for those frustrating first few years, I must admit I sometimes resented the monumental upheaval of parenthood.

But finally the first day of kindergarten—that long-awaited day of liberation!—dawned for us. Down the sidewalk we walked, hand-in-hand to the school, the bright September sun virtually igniting Evan's blond head as he shouldered his Thomas-the-Tank-Engine backpack.

When we arrived at school, Evan hesitated for a moment at the top of the steps leading down to the playground. In front of him, kids dashed about, whistles screeched, buses roared in, waves of shrieking and shouting deafened us. It was overwhelming. Then, an indelible image—Evan stepped off and, in a moment, he was gone. Not a wave, not even a backward glance. Without warning, the glorious moment turned gut-wrenching. Tears blinded me. "Where is he?" I pleaded with my husband. "Where is he? I can't see him!"

My husband took a photo of Evan and me disappearing down the sidewalk that day. When we got our photos back, I impatiently tore open the pack, eager to relive that poignant mother-and-son moment.

But when I got to the photo, I felt sick. What I saw had nothing to do with my son, and everything to do with my backside. It seemed to blot out everything else in the photo. Suddenly, I saw myself for what I was: an overweight, middle-aged mom whose size 16s weren't hiding anything.

This time, my tears were for myself. "How can this possibly be me?" I cried. I tore up the photo, as if it were that easy to destroy a memory.

Even with this heartache, I let another year go by. Half-day kindergarten doesn't liberate you the way you imagine it will. But with the coming of first grade—full days of school!—I at last had six hours to myself and I worked prodigiously, back to my old habits. A few months into the school year, however, a friend offered me a two-week guest membership to her gym.

At first, I balked. I was so eager just to keep working. But, miraculously, a niggling idea wormed its way to the fore. I thought: What if I apply my newfound knowledge of a mother's day to the dilemma of weight loss? Nix the all-out attack. Forget the daily progress check. Be content with 15 minutes here, 15 minutes there. Commit myself to the ragged, uneven—but possibly upward—path. Could it all add up?

With the barest amount of hope and curiosity, I agreed to go with my friend, still certain that I wouldn't be able to maintain a long-term interest in this enterprise. Yet inwardly I suspected this might be my only hope of conquering a battle that I'd been fighting my entire life.

I thought about what I'd do once I entered this alien place called a gym. I'd never set foot in one, had even scorned those deluded gym rats who wasted their time and money improving their bodies while their minds went to mush. Finally, I pulled a swimsuit out of my closet. At least I wouldn't have to sweat that way.

I began swimming laps three times a week. At first, it was slow going. I dragged myself to the gym. Once there, I swam in fits and starts, bored, easily tired, in a constant argument with myself. The seniors in surrounding lanes lapped me easily. Lifeguards made for the nearest chair, equipment at the ready. Once, a friend knifing through the water in full Speedo regalia shouted over, "Don't give up!" just when I thought I was doing pretty well.

And yet, four years later, it has added up. I've dropped 30 pounds and am three dress sizes smaller, even somewhat muscular. Buying my latest swimsuit, I felt almost dizzy taking size 10s into the dressing room.

The lightness extends to my mood, too. I have a new relationship with food. It's not the enemy anymore. I'm not the enemy.

I haven't dramatically changed my diet—no weighing, measuring or counting—but gradually I found myself eager to eat better, to pay attention to the signals of my body. I eat when I'm hungry and stop before I'm full. I've embraced thoughts that power me through the cravings: I know what this tastes like and I'm sure I'll have it again, so I don't need to have it right now. Or, this one: A salad tackles hunger just as well as a piece of cake does. Yet I enjoy snacks and desserts almost every day, simply choosing one or the other and having only a small amount.

Still, I'd like to swim away a few more pounds.

"Moms have a lot of fat," my now wiser fifth-grader says. Yes, my sweet boy, they do. But we can lose it, I've found. Like you, I just stepped off.

~Nancy B. Kennedy

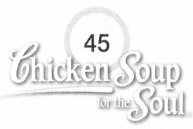

45

Something Different

Even if you fall flat on your face at least you are moving forward.

~Sue Luke

For years, I belonged to a health club and never got near the exercise machines. I went straight to the pool and swam laps, as I'd been doing since I was a teenager. I didn't understand the machines. I didn't know how to use them. They looked boring to me.

Then I took a class in creativity. "Each week do something you aren't good at," the teacher challenged. I had carefully orchestrated my weeks to be filled with things I was reasonably good at. Was I short-circuiting my own creative spirit?

I decided to start working out. I went to the upper floor of my health club, where the variety of machines and weights intimidated me. I didn't know where to start, so I hired a personal trainer to show me what to do.

"You're going to love this," the perky blonde told me. "You'll get used to it quickly and you'll love the results."

I bounced right into her enthusiasm, envisioning myself with subtly muscled arms and calves, a washboard belly and a narrower waist. I would get a pair of those leathery fingerless gloves the serious lifters wear: I would get a new workout outfit, something sexier than my XL T-shirt and ancient blue sweatpants. She showed me a series of machines sprinkled throughout the room.

"You adjust the weight here. You sit like this, make sure your arms move like this, keep your back straight, put your seat all the way back to get the maximum benefit." She instructed me on each machine and I wrote down everything she said.

"Yes!" I thought when we finished. I already felt stronger and more creative.

"No!" I thought the next morning, when I arrived at the health club, ready to whisk through my transformational routine alone. I did not recognize my machines among the multitudes. I couldn't adjust the weights. I couldn't move the seats. I couldn't remember when I kept my back straight and when I arched.

Then I remembered my creativity assignment: try something you are not good at.

Well, at least I was doing something right.

I showed a woman my instructions and she pointed me to one of my machines. A man stopped and showed me how to press in a knob so I could easily change the weights. Another woman showed me how to get the seat the right height. After 10 minutes, I was exhausted, as much from stress as from physical exertion.

"Ten more minutes," I told myself. I did 15 and felt enormously proud.

I had found five of the 12 machines and I still felt good about myself.

Patience, humility, a willingness to display below average competency and an openness to asking for help—those are just a few of the life lessons I learned those first months from working out. Plus, I got slightly firmer arms and legs.

Now I am learning free weights. My arms ache. My form is laughable. I take my puny five-pound weights over to a far corner of the gym, so the muscle men lifting barbells won't see me. I lift each weight awkwardly and as I practice I feel strong, inside and out.

~Deborah Shouse

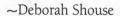

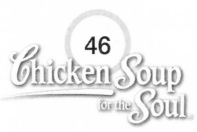

46

The Price
of a Pound of Flesh

There is just one life for each of us: our own.
~Euripedes

What was it that brought me to the brink of paying an exercise guru to whip me into shape? What made me even consider paying more per pound of body weight to lose it than I pay for groceries? And, more to the point, what snapped me out of it?

I'd gained weight the last couple of years before I retired. Instead of exercising after school, I'd gone home to my laptop where my writing and photography held me captive. I focused on what I would do when I stopped working, and I started setting things in place for a freelance writing and photography business.

I'll lose weight when I retire, I told myself. Until recently, I'd always been active—walking, biking, and working out at the gym. I had visions of my retired self leaping enthusiastically out of bed when the sun did, and going for brisk morning walks. In case of rain, there was always the exercise bike in the spare bedroom. When I don't have to get up for work, I'll want to get up, I thought.

But alas, my biorhythms had other plans. Without my alarm to rouse me, I slumbered on into midmorning. There was the new luxury of two leisurely cups of morning coffee while reading the newspaper and checking e-mail. And there was the pleasure of reading well past midnight, knowing I didn't have to drag myself out of bed to get to work the next day.

My days in retirement mode were surprisingly full. I did what I had to do, and did what I wanted to do, and kept postponing exercise to later in the day—I'll do it after lunch. I'll do it after the library. I'll do it after a nap—until eventually the day ended and I'd done nothing active. I'd climb into bed promising to get out and walk tomorrow.

My husband is the rise-and-shine get-it-over-and-done-with type, and for a while I went to the gym with him to use the treadmill, bike, or weights. But though I had risen, I never shined. The schedule—a morning one—was his, and it didn't fit me. He rushed me and I held him back. After a while, I watched him go out the door in the morning—he, clad in sweats; I, still in my bathrobe.

I puttered through two years of retirement trying to convince myself that walking on photography jaunts with my camera was "good enough" exercise, and that I'd settle into an exercise routine eventually.

So when a flyer arrived in my mail announcing a new fitness center, I hoped it would be the answer. It was a slick promotional ad designed to bring potential customers into the fitness center where the soft sell of the glossy brochure would morph into a solid sales pitch delivered by a hard-bodied recruiter.

I was curious to know the cost of the program, and they wouldn't tell me on the phone, so I checked out the facility in person. I'm a tough sell, and wasn't worried that I'd get pushed into anything my pocketbook couldn't support.

The center provided one-on-one fitness training—a private hour and a half with a personal trainer three times a week, a nutritional program, and body fat analysis. I'd visited this place four years ago to write a feature article for a newspaper, so I knew how they operated—and that they were pricy. After the grand tour and a number of questions designed to get me to admit my failures and commit myself to a trainer, my guide finally got to the bottom line.

"How much do you think this program is worth?"

"Well, I remember it was a lot four years ago, but…" I said.

"How much?"

"Oh, I don't remember the exact…"

"What would you say if I told you $2,300 for three months?"

"Goodbye."

Angus strip roast was on sale at the supermarket for $8.99 per pound and boneless chicken breasts for $4.99 a pound. According to my calculations, if I trained three times a week at the fitness center my flesh would be worth about $150 per pound.

Part of me would have liked to plunk down the money, obey orders, and emerge buff and fit in 12 weeks. I'd be lighter, but so would my bank account, and I knew from experience that it wasn't losing weight that would be the problem; it would be sustaining the loss. I needed something that would fit into my life for the long haul, something I could incorporate seamlessly into everyday life, something simpler—and cheaper.

The solution presented itself when I stopped trying to fit my round self into a square hole, when I stopped trying to reinvent myself—a miserable, if not impossible, task. When I worked with myself, not against my style. I accepted some things about myself:

1. I'm not a morning person; never was, never will be, as much as I might wish to be.
2. I need a hard and fast schedule, or I'll drift along doing what I want, quite contentedly ignoring the "shoulds" my brain nags me to do.
3. I need variety; I become easily bored with the same old thing. Even the pleasure of a morning walk would become dull.

I happily do all of the things I want or need to do during the day without the inner voice chiding constantly, "When are you going to exercise?" Because now I know when.

Come 5 p.m., I'm wearing workout clothes and heading to the gym for an exercise class—a different one each day: Pilates, step, spinning, kickboxing, muscle toning, or a dance class. My needs are met: a set schedule for a variety of classes later in the day. I work up a sweat, releasing endorphins into my bloodstream that silence my inner nag. The slow and steady pace is effective for losing weight, and more importantly in maintaining the loss. It's become a part of my day, one that I look forward to.

Recently I sat on a stationary bike in spinning class, sweating and chatting with the panting woman next to me. We were discussing our exercise routines.

"Man, when I retire I'm going to spend all day at the gym," she said.

I didn't share the mental journey that had landed me on the bike next to hers that evening. She'll make her own discoveries when she retires.

I simply said, "That's not my style."

When it comes to exercising, or anything else in life, to thine own self be true — right down to the biorhythms.

~Ruth Douillette

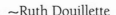

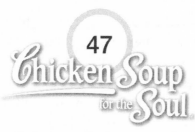

47

A Healthy New Mantra

Attitude is a little thing that makes a big difference.
~Winston Churchill

His spare leg slung over his shoulder, Denny saunters into the gym. He flashes his 100-watt smile at my husband Bart and me, as we chat idly beside an exercise bike—just a couple of 50-somethings hoping to work off the effects of desk jobs, stress, and our love for food, wine and beer.

I'm no athlete but I like to stay fit. A number of wonderful instructors have inspired me over the years, in my varied program of yoga, Pilates, kettle bells, and cardio.

But for my husband, there has been only one influential trainer: Dennis Chipollini. Before he started working out with Denny a few years ago, my husband was discouraged. Embarrassed about his weak upper body and concerned about his lack of energy, he wanted to tone up and lose weight. As his wife, I agreed, and worried that "I'm tired" was becoming his mantra.

His usual workout regimen, mostly cardiovascular exercises like spinning and walking, wasn't working. He knew he needed more, so he decided to add weight training with a personal trainer.

But sticking to his commitment was hard. Some mornings I heard Bart groan, "I don't feel like working out." But he went anyway. After a while, I noticed the muscles in his shoulders, the way his jeans fit. I liked the changes I saw. Bart explained, "When you exercise with Denny, you can't get away with excuses, because Denny can do more with one leg than most people can with two."

So when my husband suggested I join him and Denny for a Saturday morning workout a few months ago, I eagerly agreed. I wanted to meet the man who inspires my husband to keep on exercising.

Denny adjusts the weight on the squat-lift machine, towering over me, his tank top showing off his strong biceps, his gym shorts revealing his prosthetic left leg. This leg, the one with the picture of Betty Boop, is named Betty. "I name all my legs," Denny says. "I've got about nine of them."

Amid the clanking of weights and whirring of treadmills, Denny puts us through our paces. Twenty squat-lifts, three laps, 20 squat-lifts, three laps. As I circle the track, one foot in front of the other, I think of Denny's remarkable story, how on a rainy morning in 1989, his car hydroplaned and slammed into a guardrail. "BAM!" Denny supplies the sound effects. "Wow! That was close," he remembered thinking with relief. Then he looked down. Both of his legs had been severed.

Pain overtook him, but Denny wasn't ready for death. He was just beginning his life—his wife Sue was expecting their first child. He knew he had to stop the bleeding. "I was pinned under the steering wheel. I couldn't move—but I could use my mind. I visualized myself in a hospital, doctors working to save me. I willed myself to be calm, and the bleeding slowed down. At that moment I learned the incredible power of the human mind."

He endured months in the hospital and 15 surgeries to save his legs. In the midst of one operation, in the same hospital, Sue gave birth to their son, Nicholas.

Physicians saved his right foot, but not the left leg. "You're never going to walk again," one doctor told him.

"You wanna bet?" Denny said.

The day of his accident, Denny learned the power of the mind. He used that knowledge to create his own rehab. While Sue worked to support them, he dragged himself upstairs to lift weights. Ten months after that doctor's prediction, Denny was walking with a cane. Three years after that, he ran his first 5K race. "They said I wouldn't walk again." That 100-watt grin flashes again. "They didn't say anything about running."

With Denny's coaching, my "new improved" husband lifts weights he thought he'd never even budge. Twenty squat-lifts, three laps, 20 squat-lifts, three laps. My quads burn, but if Denny can run a 5K with a smile on his face, how can I complain?

After that first race, Denny remembers, a young boy told him, "Mister, you're my hero." Denny recognized that an amputee who runs marathons gets attention, and that attention could be harnessed. He just didn't know yet what he was meant to harness it for.

At the gym, my husband and I flail our arms and legs in a clumsy attempt at abdominal exercises on the mat. Denny calls out, "C'mon! What are you guys doing?"

Bart laughs but we try harder.

People call Denny a hero, but Denny's hero is his son Nicholas, now a fine young man in his 20s, who has neurofibromatosis, which causes tumors on nerve endings, as well as autism and Tourette's syndrome. When Denny and Sue learned the kids were excluding Nicholas at school, Denny discovered his true calling—to use the attention he attracts to inspire and educate. This part of the story resonates with Bart and me, because we have a son and nephew who also face challenges.

So Denny founded Generation Hope, an organization that raises understanding about disabilities. To publicize his cause, Denny speaks to rapt audiences of all ages, telling his story, repeating his message of acceptance, and his mantra, "No excuses, no limits." He has competed in triathlons, as well as full and half marathons. He bicycled across Pennsylvania. He became the first person to carry both the Olympic and Paralympic torches. "My amputation is my gift," I've heard Denny say. "I wear it like a badge of courage."

"Okay," Denny commands, setting the timer on his watch. "Three-minute plank!" Bart and I drop to a push-up position. "No saggy butts." Denny falls to the mat and pikes up into a perfect plank.

Denny advocates Positive Psychology, nutrition, chia seed, good wine and Dogfish Head beer. He projects a positive attitude, but admits there have been dark, private moments when the support of his wife and kids got him through, including his ordeal with Hepatitis C, which he contracted from a blood transfusion. "I don't know how they put up with me!" he laughs, shaking his head. "When you're down, it's the little gesture—the 'human touch'—that gets you back."

Right about now, my abs burn and my elbows are sweating. I don't think I can hold the plank one nanosecond longer. But there's Denny, right beside us, smiling. And maybe that's what keeps Bart—and now, me—coming back. A positive attitude, the high of overcoming personal obstacles—and the human touch.

"Next time I set the timer!" Bart laughs.

"Whatsa matter? Tired?"

Suddenly I realize—I haven't heard Bart say, "I'm tired" in months. Now that he's got more energy, he's swapped that old mantra for a healthy new one: "No excuses, no limits." Still in my plank position, I beam with pride.

The timer beeps. Whew! I flop onto the mat. "That's it, you guys!" Denny sings out, "Go have breakfast!"

~Faith Paulsen

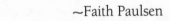

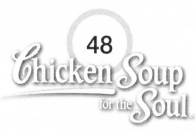

48

She Called Me Olga

*The greatest pleasure in life
is doing what people say you cannot do.*

~Bagehot

Junior high school was my undoing when it came to many things, but especially my fitness and my self-esteem. My gym teacher took to calling me Olga, after Olga Korbut, the gold medal gymnast. I can still hear her sarcastic tone when she told me it was my turn to do my gymnastic routine. I was an ungainly girl, tall and clumsy, and let's just say that once I survived the year, I gave up on sports. My self-confidence was so destroyed that I didn't realize that I was in fact a good swimmer, volleyball player and bicyclist. I thought that I was hopeless and I did everything I could to avoid exercise and athletics. I considered myself lucky my senior year when I became so ill from mononucleosis that I was excused from gym class for the rest of the year.

The years passed. I managed to avoid the intramural games at my college and never bothered to find the beautiful gymnasium. I never participated in the softball games in my town or in the parent/child swim meets. Once in a while, I joined exercise classes, but never was successful. And then, one day, I found myself in my 40s, overweight, out-of-shape and miserable. I had just spoken to my doctor, who had given me my recent results and they were dire.

I realized that I was in a now or never situation and so, without telling anyone, I summoned up all my courage and drove to the nearest gym. I walked up to the desk and said that I wanted to join immediately. The woman was surprised that I hadn't asked for a tour or inquired about the price. To be honest, I was afraid that I was going to give up again, and I just wanted to commit immediately. I couldn't even get started that day because I had neglected to wear exercise clothes and sneakers.

The next morning, I drove back to the gym and forced myself to go inside. I was nervous about learning to use the machines and about looking like a fraud in my workout clothes. Fortunately, as soon as I entered, I saw a woman who had been a sports teacher for my younger daughter. Bonnie was welcoming and showed me how to use some of the machines. That morning, I managed five minutes on the elliptical, and if it hadn't been for her kind encouragement, I wouldn't have lasted a minute.

I went to the gym almost every day. I tried not to make a schedule. I just went whenever I possibly could. And every day I did whatever I could do, and then maybe a little more. Bonnie helped me, always smiling and showing me another routine. I finally got up the courage to stop taking all of her time and to hire a "real" trainer. I told him how afraid I was, and about my junior high school teacher. He told me that it was time to move on, and he was right. With his guidance, I became stronger and healthier.

It's three years later, and now I'm one of the regulars at the gym, someone who everyone knows. I try to go every morning, and some mornings, when I really don't feel like going, I go anyway. Every day I do what I think I can do and then a little bit more. I see my friends and still enjoy working out with Bonnie. Lately we've been doing spin classes together. It amazes me every time that I can keep up. I'm not going to lie and say that I've lost a tremendous amount of weight and am now a size 2. I'm a middle-aged woman and I've come to face certain realities. I will never become a size 2, but what I have become is more important than that. Finally, after many years of avoiding exercise, I've made it a priority in my life. I'm healthier and happier than I've ever been, certainly more than I was in junior high school.

Take that, Miss D—!

~Lisa Coll Nicolaou

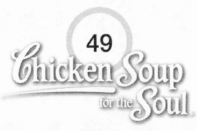

49

Pool Walking

The water is your friend.
You don't have to fight with water,
just share the same spirit as the water,
and it will help you move.
~Aleksandr Popov

Sitting on the edge of my bed, I contemplated how to approach day one of my Twenty-Eight-Days-to-a-New-You. Barely able to stand with my sore back, I hesitantly pulled on my sweatpants. I breathed deeply. In through my nose. Out through my mouth. I knew I had to keep today's appointment. Tuesday was my day off and having to reschedule this engagement would only postpone the initiation of my healthy new lifestyle.

A few weeks prior, my husband made a decision for us—we were going to become members of our local fitness center, The Club, and we were joining that day! For years, when my husband, Anthony, brought up this idea I balked at the enrollment fee and the prospect of committing to monthly membership dues. After all, he's a runner; can't running be done for free and outside? With strong gusts of wind and a winter storm warning in the news, Anthony simply said, "We're doing it."

I'm not naive. I know exercising provides great health benefits, energizes all life forces and even helps people shrink a few sizes. Although this is what most people want, some of us (me) are not quite able to make the connection of how it applies to us. Of course we want the "endorphin high." We simply prefer to achieve it another way. Lying across the couch, devouring a bowl of popcorn, and watching *Guiding Light* provided me with the perfect endorphin trifecta. Sedentary meets utopia. Through no doing of my own, my comfort level was about to shift.

At The Club, Shirley, the skinny-as-a-swizzle-stick membership coordinator greeted us. Pleasant enough in her skin-tight black skirt and *Sex and the City* pumps, Shirley spoke to Anthony and me during a club tour. Ms. Shirley had her homily down pat. Traveling this maze, we learned the 40,000 square foot sports club offered an array of state-of-the-art fitness equipment, a weight room, racquetball courts, classes such as kickboxing and Pilates, an Olympic size pool and a bullpen of personal trainers. My sleepwalking ended when I heard "…a sauna, steam room, Jacuzzi, and locker rooms complete with toiletries, including free disposable razors." Our victory lap crossed the finish line at Shirley's desk with the signing of many membership papers and a hefty check—no pun intended.

Slugging back to our car carrying The Club's membership folder and free water bottle, Anthony sensed my horror at having committed myself to a life of exercise. He kindly suggested, "Why don't you set up a meeting with one of the personal trainers to discuss your goals? This way you'll know where to begin." I was left with no choice but to nod.

So here I sat on this gray February morning in excruciating pain determined to get this appointment over with. With heroic effort I kept my 9:00 a.m. appointment; unfortunately, my new personal trainer did not. "Are you kidding me?" I thought. "Have I been stood up, when I can't even stand up?"

The Club's athletic director, Jerry, was mortified to learn one of his trainers forgot about a new client. "I'm really sorry about this Mrs. Molinaro; I see your appointment is in the book. I'm not sure how the mix-up occurred."

Hunched over the reception desk with my bad back, I leaned in and whispered, "Jerry, it's really okay. Postponing this consultation is actually better for me today. I injured my back and am more than willing to reschedule. Obviously, I can barely stand straight and shouldn't have even come here today."

Either Jerry couldn't hear me or he wasn't buying my story, because he switched into search and rescue mode. Jerry was finding me a trainer and The Club would reign! My stomach knotted. Oh, how I wished I had had the guts to cancel.

In order for Lynda, "my fueled by Red Bull personal trainer," to develop the most effective exercise program for me, she asked a series of questions about my current fitness level and personal goals. Are you experiencing stress? When was the last time you exercised? Perched on a stool near the juice bar (for easy access should I need a banana smoothie), my only obligation was to answer her honestly. Throughout the hour, Lynda repeatedly responded to my monosyllabic answers with, "No problem, my mother doesn't exercise either." I warmly smiled. The second time she said this, I responded by raising my eyebrows and pursing my lips. How old did this twit think I was? By the tenth reference to her mother, I began rocking back and forth. Gym people have no soul. I hated her. I wanted out!

We slowly moved our meet-and-greet to a tiny dimly lit interrogation room so Lynda could weigh me. This was an entrapment. Hearing her broadcast "the number," I began silently praying, "Please let me be one of those women who is weeks away from giving birth, yet had no idea she was pregnant."

Finally, Lynda finished her initial assessment and assigned me my first exercise regime. "Walk in the pool," she prescribed. "Walk in the pool?" I repeated in disbelief. Didn't she know I couldn't stand up straight and that I would have to wear a bathing suit in the pool? I felt like the 500-pound person they discovered in some apartment building on the ninth floor. She gave me a death stare. I stared back. The room chilled. That settled it. I was going pool walking.

Humbled, I returned later in the week for my sanctioned hour of pool walking. Sergeant Lynda provided handheld pool weights and a kickboard. The water was freezing. I walked forward, backward, and sideways. I grabbed the kickboard and swam a few laps. Within the hour my trainer was teaching me squatting and stretching exercises.

My body was actually sweating. The water became tepid. After a few weeks of pool walking I got up the courage to attend a water aerobics class. I loved it! Years later, I still look forward to the Tuesday and Thursday morning classes, where women just like me edge into the pool and start walking!

What started out begrudgingly as a Twenty-Eight-Day journey to a new me, led to a three-year voyage of self-discovery—and a 15- to 20-pound weight loss (accepting fluctuation is a learned virtue). If by making simple food choices (not every sandwich requires cheese), moving more (I got out of my own way) and complaining less (the first step to grasping the endorphin high), this soap opera-watching woman was able to simply do it, anyone can... sometimes all we need is to be thrown in the deep end!

~Beth A. Molinaro

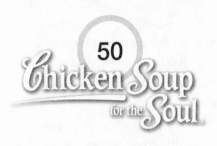

50

Sweat Sisters

Help one another, is part of the religion of sisterhood.
~Louisa May Alcott

I've said it before, and I'll say it again: I'll never love exercising. I do it because I know I should. I do it faithfully while my resolve is strong, and not so faithfully when it falters. And truth to tell, since I began a regular gym routine a few years ago, I do feel stronger and more fit.

But when I miss a few days, I don't miss the crunches or leg stretches or working my glutes. I definitely don't yearn to be doing the lateral lifts that exhaust me.

What I miss is the companionship of my fellow gym members—all women.

I almost joined one of those gyms where the bodies were sleek and the men and women seemed utterly comfortable together as they worked those pecs. But I fled after a trial run.

I felt mortified by my own klutziness, embarrassed by how uncoordinated I was and how many years older I was than the young things who could run for hours on the treadmills—and talk on their cell phones at the same time.

But I'm safe and comfortable in this world of women of all ages and ranges of dexterity, where the conversation is part of the fun.

I know you're not supposed to go to the gym for your social sustenance, but when you work alone at home as I do most days, just getting out into the world is a treat. And being with women who get to know one another not even by name, but by the color of their T-shirts, is often my "recess."

By now, we know one another's habits.

Linda, the adorable, spirited home economics teacher, is dogged. She not only does the circuit—she also does the stepper. Her good nature is infectious.

Sue is gentle and quiet, always gracious, and graceful on machines that make me feel like a person on a bender.

Hope lives up to her name, with a steadfast and upbeat approach to the workout.

Our conversations roam from politics to fashion to vitamins. Some of us take them faithfully. Others think they're a waste of money.

On the walls around us are quotations, word games to ponder as we sweat, posters to keep us inspired and motivated.

But it's the steady conversational flow that seems to keep us doing the "dip shrugs" that work our deltoids and dorsal muscles.

Most of us are married. Or getting married.

I spent my last visit talking to Lauren, the slender young bride-to-be, about her gown, her attendants' gowns, which are the rich color of cinnamon, and about whether she'll wear her hair up or down.

It made the time go so quickly that I was almost disappointed when I'd finished the circuit.

Woman-talk is rich and textured. It's curious how it ebbs and flows, but it always does.

On most days, I leave the gym with a new thought, a new recipe, or an idea I didn't arrive with.

Occasionally, I leave feeling sad or worried about someone whose name I may not know, but who is clearly having a rough spell.

I was thrilled when one of our members finished treatment for a serious illness, and was back among us, restored and ready for her workout. I was touched by her resilience and her great joy in just being able to resume the routine.

I love hearing Pam's views on the latest plays. She's informed and smart and ready to try new theatrical experiences. I'm not nearly as brave in my choices.

And if truth be told, I'm glad that there are no men to change the mood. I have absolutely nothing against men, but at the gym, I love the feeling of a sisterhood, a mutual support group.

So three days a week, I pull up to the place where I have sisters-in-sweat. With them, I grumble about my kids, my work, the electrician who stood me up, my husband's driving.

And somehow, in less than an hour, I'm feeling better. And stronger. And so virtuous.

When I leave, I tell them that I'll be back soon.

And the amazing thing is that even though I hate to exercise, I always return.

~Sally Schwartz Friedman

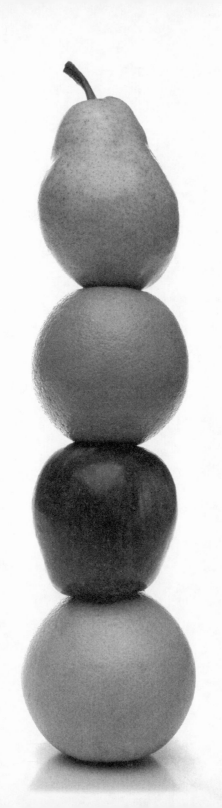

Chapter 6

Shaping the New You

Liking Myself

*Whenever I find something to criticize about myself—
I will follow with a positive thought about myself.*

~Richard Simmons, The Book of Hope

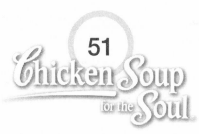

51

Ready to Listen

What I need is someone
who will make me do what I can.
~Ralph Waldo Emerson

Today, I weigh nearly 150 pounds less than I did three years ago, and the weight loss began with a compliment: "You look great."

I was the mother of two adopted special needs children when I decided to go back to college. Our daughter was beginning college herself, our son doing well after years of struggling, when something inside me whispered, "It's time." I hadn't made myself a priority for over a decade. I had no idea that not only would I finish my degree and go on to grad school, but I would also lose 150 pounds in the process!

My weight had climbed as my self-confidence sank under the strain of being the mother of two wonderful yet challenged children. Often I didn't feel as if I had the answers, and I worried I was failing at everything. Before long, I was 180 pounds over my ideal weight, and I felt food was the only bright spot in my life. The troubles with our children had caused my beloved husband and me often to feel disconnected from one another.

One day after I returned to college, I dressed in a suit for an appointment with the head of the English department to discuss my senior research project, and the professor not only noticed, but also commented upon it. I'm sure it was quite a change from the stretchy jeans and T-shirts I habitually wore to class. "You look great," he said, and I realized then that I wasn't invisible. That day I went home and purged my wardrobe of the most hated pieces of "fat" clothing. I vowed to rebuild it slowly with only clothes I would be proud to be seen wearing. If this professor I so respected was letting me know the way to get ahead in my career was to look professional, I would listen.

"I don't look great," I thought when he said that, looking down, "but I bet I could." I had already let him challenge my mind with books, so I decided to allow that compliment to challenge me to attain my physical best. I had never been thin, and I could blame it on genetics. I didn't exactly look out of place in family photos. But I was ready for the challenge. I had used his advice to improve my writing and my critical thinking skills, and I saw the connection between developing my brain and my body for the first time.

I began to exercise, slowly at first. I did Denise Austin videos (20 minutes each) every morning. I took walks when the weather was nice. I once again tried low-carb eating, which quickly took care of my cravings, and virtually eliminated my need for nightly mindless eating fests. I began to read or write instead of watching television, and bit by bit, the weight came off. I went to a nutritionist when I felt I was backsliding a bit, just to be sure I stayed the course. I also entered and won a weight loss competition at work; having my picture put in the local paper for the win was a blast for a former chunky. I felt fantastic!

I committed more and more time to exercise. I would like to lose another 30 pounds, but I have kept my weight within a 10-pound range for the past year and a half, and I can't imagine I could ever feel better than I do right now. I am a size 12-14, and I feel alive and hopeful, as if I could do anything. Most days I exercise for two hours—an hour in the morning, and a relaxing walk in the evening, or I lift weights while watching TV with my husband. I have discovered I adore exercise, and I might even enter a race at some point. Who knew?

I still eat low-carb when my weight begins to creep up, but mostly I listen to my body and eat what it wants, while striving to focus on healthier foods such as whole grains and fresh produce. I still struggle to fit in vegetables, as my taste buds don't always agree with my body on that one! I also try to get three servings of dairy a day, as well as eight or more glasses of water. Sometimes we try to reinvent the wheel when the wheel's rolling just fine—the conventional wisdom about eating less and moving more really works!

At my son's graduation party, I publicly ate two pieces of ice cream cake without a trace of guilt. If I really want it, I eat it. Life is long, and losing weight and keeping it off will be an ongoing project. That's the only way to approach it.

For the first time in my life, I feel attractive. I am able to look back, too, and see the love and care I put into raising my children. Maybe I didn't have all the answers, but they know I love them, and they are striving for their goals, too, as they see me go towards mine. Losing weight is only the first of many goals—right now I am writing my first novel. If I can lose weight, I can do anything! My husband, while delighted that his wife now gets wolf whistles, has made it clear he will love me whatever my size. We have been able to reconnect as my self-confidence has returned.

As for that professor who gave me the confidence to begin my weight loss—while I did the work, he gave me the courage to begin. He had no way of knowing that those three small words spoken on a random Wednesday morning would transform a life.

~Drema Sizemore Drudge

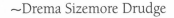

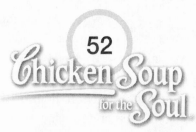

52

Climbing
Nevis Peak

Self-conquest is the greatest of victories.
~Plato

My trips to the Caribbean usually include nothing but sun, sand, and umbrella drinks. But on a recent getaway to the West Indies my husband, Tom, and I ventured out of our comfort zones and climbed to the top of Nevis Peak, a dormant volcano in the center of Nevis, a small island nation located about 220 miles southeast of Puerto Rico.

We had spent our honeymoon in Nevis and had admired the beauty of the Peak but gave no thought to visiting the summit. In the weeks leading up to our return—to celebrate our fifth anniversary—we discussed climbing the mountain, though neither of us had ever attempted such a feat.

On our first full day in Nevis, we arranged a guide through the concierge at the Four Seasons. Early the next morning we met our guide, Sheldon, and traveled together by taxi to the staging point for the climb.

The hike started out pretty much as we'd imagined—a moderately uphill nature walk. We passed old, delightfully rundown sugar mills, breadfruit and banana trees, and mischievous green vervet monkeys that made us laugh.

"No need for dat, mon," said Sheldon, as I slathered my arm with sunscreen. "We'll be out of da sun in a few." Wearing Dickies and a green logo T-shirt, his style screamed urban hipster, not mountain guide, and his thick Caribbean accent made his words dance.

He was right. Minutes later the forest began to close in on us and the sun was gone. We were dwarfed by the colossal roots and towering trees as we made our way through the dark, dense, and muddy jungle. The incline continued to increase until it seemed impossible to walk without falling off the earth. That's when we encountered the first knotted rope, needed to aid our ascent, followed by dozens more. Hours passed; my heart raced and drops of sweat made my eyes sting. As I continuously climbed over rocks, maneuvered under fallen trees and used the rope to pull myself up nearly vertical slopes, it dawned on me—I had the strength to do so, because for most of my life, I wouldn't have been able to.

Thanks to my general lethargy, combined with my love for ice cream and almost daily dates with jumbo bags of Doritos, I hit my all-time high of 216 pounds during my sophomore year of college. All the nacho cheese flavor and Cherry Garcia in the world couldn't mask the shame I felt for letting my body pass the 200-pound mark. It took a nasty fall in which I severely sprained my ankle to change my ways. The fall forced me into six weeks of physical therapy to help strengthen my ankle. Ultimately, the fall and subsequent stint of PT were blessings in disguise. I discovered my body related really well to exercise and, much to my dismay, I relished working up a sweat.

And now, here I was, 65 pounds thinner and climbing a mountain; making my body work harder than any other time in my life. Even after my significant weight loss and ability to kick it out in a spinning class, I still didn't think of myself as fit. But after reaching the cloud-covered summit and making our trek back down the mountain, I changed the way I thought about my body—physically powerful and beautiful.

As we approached the edge of the jungle, it began to rain. The light drizzle turned to torrential downpour and I felt an overwhelming sense of cleanliness. The mud that by now covered every inch of my body washed away, as did the negative feelings about myself that I'd harbored for years.

~Jennifer Leckstrom

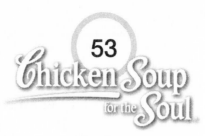

53

My Transformation

*Living a healthy lifestyle will only deprive you
of poor health, lethargy, and fat.*

~Jill Johnson

Oprah talks about that "ah ha moment," something that changes you forever. Mine came when my mother-in-law sent me pictures that she'd taken at Christmas. The first two were of my beautiful sons opening Christmas gifts. The third one was of my husband standing next to an old, heavy-set woman. At first I thought who is that old lady? No one had visited besides my in-laws, and then it hit me like someone had poured a bucket of ice water over me. I was that fat, old lady. I was posed in the picture eating a double helping of peanut butter pie. My first thought was, boy, I could really go for a piece of that pie. My second thought was, gee, I look terrible. I sank in my chair and burst into tears. Something needed to be done.

Throughout my life I had gone through transformations. In high school I was average looking, didn't really stand out, but something happened in my mid-20s. I had a nice shape and a somewhat pretty face. I noticed that men were attracted to me. I certainly wasn't a super model by any means, but I felt good about myself when I looked in the mirror.

Then came marriage, two children mixed with aging, and weight gain. I didn't feel desirable anymore. All I felt was disgust and a dislike for who I'd become. I knew what to do but instead of doing it, I turned to food. There is no magic pill when it comes to losing weight. And it certainly isn't going to happen in a few weeks. It takes time and patience. It's hard work.

For some crazy reason I've always enjoyed running. I'm not a long distance runner, probably two or three miles a day. I also know about resistance weight training. I also know what foods to put into my body: the whole grains, fruits, vegetables, fish, chicken, and the good fats found in walnuts and olive oil. My problem was pulling it all together.

After my "ah ha moment" I developed a healthy weight loss plan. The days I don't have to work I'm on the treadmill at 7:30 a.m. I don't even think about it. I just do it. The days I have to work, I'm on the treadmill at 3:30 p.m. I do 300 sit-ups a day. And every other day I lift free weights for about 20 minutes. A few nights a week, there's tennis and basketball with the kids.

I also found a connection between God and food while I turned my body into something healthy that I could be proud of again. One day for a split second in the grocery store I was tempted to pile my cart with desserts and ice cream. But it quickly passed and I found myself drawn toward the greens and reds in the vegetable aisle. I felt close to God. It was like he was telling me, "I made all this food for you. Please don't turn your back on it; please, don't fill your body with junk. Make yourself healthy." I shoved some broccoli into a bag and piled several sweet potatoes in my cart. It gave me a deep appreciation for God. I feel like He's the finest cook in the world, and whenever I choose a salad over processed food I'm complimenting the chef.

Pulling all of this together was not easy. I had to exercise five to six days a week, make sure the fridge was loaded with healthy food, and most importantly, break old patterns. The worst part for me was not being able to snack at night. There are a few nights a week that I will allow myself a mini bag of popcorn and one low-fat, low-sugar treat, but most nights I don't snack. At first I felt depressed. It was like I lost my best friend. I mean, who doesn't want their best buddy, the chocolate chip ice cream bar, along when watching their favorite TV show? But I wouldn't allow myself to go there, and if I couldn't control my urges then I just wouldn't watch TV. I learned two important things: food is not my best friend—I am—and sometimes you must give up something to get something better in return. Slowly the weight started to drop, and as more came off, I not only looked better, but felt better, too.

When I made the commitment to lose weight, I also made a commitment to write a romance novel. I've not only been struggling with my weight for the last 10 years but wanted to write, as well, so I combined the two goals. With every couple of chapters I wrote it seemed like another five pounds dropped off. By the time I was finished with the book and sent it to a publisher, I had reached my goal of losing 25 pounds. I believe that doing what I always wanted to do, writing the book, distracted me from overeating.

I remember the day I went into the store and traded my stretch pants for some cute, little white shorts. I caught a glimpse of my new figure in the mirror and started to cry. I was so proud of myself for all the hard work.

Next, came the stares. Now don't get me wrong, I'm a happily married woman, but attention from the opposite sex is flattering. One day as I was walking up my driveway, a fellow in a red pickup truck slowed down and said to his friend, "That girl is hot!" At first I didn't know who he was referring to. I looked around to see if one of my friends had stopped by. Then it dawned on me, he was talking about me. I couldn't contain my smile.

I have now entered maintenance mode. I weigh myself once a week. I choose healthy foods over junk foods. I exercise five or six days a week. If it's someone's birthday or I'm at a party, I'll indulge, but the difference is I will only have one piece of cake instead of three or four. If I've had French fries the night before, the next day I get right back on track. It's all in moderation.

Some people ask how I find the time. I made time to sit on the couch and eat; now I've replaced that habit with healthy eating and exercising. I also feel that every time I take care of myself, it's my way of thanking God for giving me a healthy and reliable body. It's my gift back to Him, and a gift I'm teaching my children, to take care of themselves.

As for my romance life with my husband, I finally feel desirable again. Things over the past few months have really started to heat up in our bedroom. And I'm not saying that because our air conditioner is on the blink again.

~Terri L. Knight

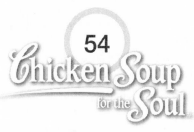

54

Eat, Exercise, Brush Your Teeth

You are your own judge.
The verdict is up to you.
~Astrid Alauda

"Y**ou have eating disorder N.O.S."** Those words came from my physician only a few days after New Year's Day several years ago. N.O.S. stands for not otherwise specified. I had a cross between anorexia and bulimia. My eating habits had been deteriorating for almost a year.

I'd grown up living a healthy lifestyle. My parents were health-conscious and emphasized the importance of eating right and exercising. Growing up, Goldfish crackers were considered a treat, and there was no soda in the house. I already had small bones and a lean body when I got mononucleosis my junior year in high school.

Normally, there is a loss of appetite with the illness, but I had an abscess in my throat, and the only time that it did not hurt was when I was eating. On top of constantly eating anything that I craved, I could not exercise due to fatigue and the risk of rupturing my spleen, which is a concern during and after having mono.

I gained 10 pounds. So once I was better I went back to exercising and eating right. The springtime came, and people were complimenting me on how great I looked. But by the end of junior year, a falling out with my group of girl friends triggered a downhill spiral. I had a hard time controlling my emotions, and struggled to deal with everything going on in my life, so I started to over-exercise and under-eat.

The summer between my junior and senior year is filled with awful memories. I was a terror to be around for my younger sister and parents. I would eat a slice of cheese, a piece of chicken, and some vegetables for a day's worth of food on top of running several miles in the middle of a hot summer day.

Some days I found myself so hungry that I couldn't think straight, yet the compliments would keep flowing. "What a great little body you have," or "you're so tiny." Those comments kept me going, along with the discovery of laxatives.

I've always had a sweet tooth, so I still found it difficult not being able to eat candy or cookies. Some days I would eat everything in sight, and before going to bed, I would take at least four laxative pills, dehydrating and emptying my body.

I thought that I was losing all the weight and calories that I had consumed, but really I was just harming my digestive tract. In the winter of my senior year, I admitted to a friend that I had been using laxatives. She didn't run and tell my parents, but her genuine concern for me helped me to stop taking them.

Finally, I broke down to my parents. It was one of the hardest things to do: admitting that I knew I had a problem, and that I wasn't this perfect person that I lead everyone to believe I was.

I began outpatient treatment at one of the top eating disorder clinics in America. I saw a therapist once a week, along with a dietician and a physician. It wasn't easy and I did relapse.

I struggled for a year and started seeing a therapist in college. My eating habits would alter based on what was going on in my life, but as I learned in therapy, eating should not correlate with emotions.

While I was seeing my therapist in high school, she said the simplest, but most profound thing to me. "Eating is like brushing your teeth. Would you wake up in the morning and not brush your teeth? No. Well it's the same thing with eating."

I've learned that, for me, sometimes if I'm stressed I'll eat more or less, but that's okay. As long as I am eating, and conscious of what is going on, I'm fine. Being aware of my body and my surroundings brought me to the place I am today.

I can now say that I have not consumed laxatives in almost four years. I am beyond proud of myself. I exercise daily, not to lose weight, but because it makes me feel good and I enjoy it. I eat balanced meals because my body actually feels better when I'm not depriving it or feeding it with junk food.

Admitting I had a problem was one part of this journey, but overcoming it has helped me learn that, no matter what is going on in my life, one always has to eat, just like one always has to brush one's teeth.

~Amanda Romaniello

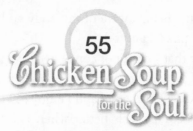

55

Wonderfully Made

To free us from the expectations of others,
to give us back to ourselves —
there lies the great, singular power of self-respect.
~Joan Didion

"My name is Thurmeka and I am fat. I would like to change that. I'm going on a diet to lose weight. I weigh 95 pounds." I wrote this on the inside cover of a book called *Don't Call Me Fatso* when I was seven years old. My stomach squirmed when I read my seven-year-old handwriting. I realized that the words I wrote then were the beginning of what I would continue to write and think about myself.

Growing up I was called chubby or "big-boned" by adults. I hated both of those words and wanted them to disappear from the English language. (What was "big-boned" anyway?) Even though I disliked the words that adults used to classify me, they were gentle compared to some of the things my peers said to me. If I got into an argument with someone they would say, "What are you going to do? Sit on me?" or "Shut up your fat self!" I used to pretend it didn't bother me, but it did. Instead of discarding the lies I heard about myself, they became my truth.

I let the fear of people's perceptions rule my life. I wore jeans and sweatshirts in the summer (including at the beach), kept my coat on in school, and only wore long skirts. My mother and I got into many arguments about this. It hurt her to see me react to my reflection in this way, but I just thought she did not understand. I knew my perception of myself was abnormal when I told my high school boyfriend he could not hug me because his arms might not fit around me and he would feel my fat. Clearly my perception of myself was distorted, but I did not see it that way at the time. It affected many relationships and I missed out on opportunities because I let fear consume me.

Throughout my college years, I tried many fad diets and came to the conclusion that my body was wired differently than any other human. I was destined to be "fat" forever. After years of thinking this way, and after many people telling me I had a problem, I sat back and evaluated what was going on. I was carrying a lot of emotional weight that was literally weighing me down. My struggle to accept myself kept me from living life. I had to realize and accept that I was wonderfully made and I had to love myself. I also had to stop comparing myself with others because I was not them; I was me!

At that time I was at my all-time high of 189 pounds. I looked at myself in the mirror and I said, "I like me." I finally pointed out the good and didn't focus on the bad. I began working out at a gym with one of my friends and we held each other accountable. I also joined kickboxing classes and dancing classes that I knew I would enjoy. Instead of looking at my eating plan as a diet, I looked upon it as the beginning of an exciting new journey. I enjoyed food instead of being afraid of it. At the end of my three-month journey I was down to 166 pounds. Even though I was not at my goal weight, I was happy. I did more than shed physical weight; I shed years of pain and loneliness. I learned how to love me and as a result I was better able to take care of myself. Now I enjoy eating healthy and exercising because it is a part of loving myself rather than a chore. I know I am beautiful on the inside and out, and my goal is to exude beauty through the way I live my life. Here is what I write now: "My name is Thurmeka and I am wonderfully made."

~Thurmeka S. Ward

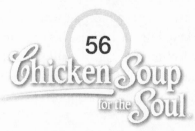

56

Taking Control of My Body Image

*Life is far too rich, interesting and short
to waste on hating your body.*
~Author Unknown

'm thirty-one and looking at photos from a recent work function. "Look at my arms," I complain to my co-worker in an instant message. "They're so chubby. No matter what I do or how thin I get."

"Genetics," she types back.

"You know what's weird?" I write. "When I was a teenager, I didn't have these kinds of body issues."

"Don't start now," she warns.

Later that day, I realize that I lied to my friend and to myself. There were so many instances of body hatred in my past, starting even before I was a teenager, and continuing, and continuing, and continuing:

I'm twelve, on vacation on Eastern Long Island with my parents and my best friend at the time, Kristina. Even then I could see that she was and would always be prettier than me—thinner, too. We walk down a beautiful, wooded road to get to the beach, wearing bikini tops and shorts. I watch her back when she walks in front of me, and I hate my body as it compares to hers. It's only years later, when I look at pictures from that trip, that I see two beautiful girls.

I'm fifteen, standing in front of my full-length mirror, getting ready to walk to my friend Stephanie's house. I've just gotten back from sleep-away camp, and this will be the first time I've seen my friends in a month. I think (and hope) some boys will be there. I wear a pink shirt that brings out the rosiness of my cheeks. I've painted my nails a similar color. I stare at my forehead, willing it to shrink. I've decided it's too long, and bangs are not in, so I can't even hide it. I wonder whether, if I could magically make an inch of it disappear, would I, if it meant that I lost an inch of height? With only 5'2" on me—another thing I hate about myself—I can't really afford to get shorter. But this forehead!

I'm sixteen and I just ate two Twix bars. Two full candy bars, meaning four caramel and chocolate-covered cookies. I feel disgusting and disgusted. I go to the bathroom and put my fingers down my throat. Before I can get them far enough in to even gag, some reflex makes me pull my fingers out of my mouth. So much for bulimia, I think.

It's the summer that I turn nineteen and I've just had my heart broken. I pull away from my friends, learning for the first time how vulnerable love makes you. I don't want to give anyone the power to hurt me. I take control of the one thing that feels within my grasp—eating. Most days I allow myself only grapefruit and saltines. Occasionally I'll eat a real meal for dinner. I don't remember hoping for weight loss, but of course I lose the 15 pounds I gained my freshman year of college. I go back to college that fall and the heartbreaker says to me, "You look amazing. It's going to be hard not to want to get back together with you." I'm so shocked, I can't think of what to say. For weeks I wonder if he broke up with me because I was fat. And did I somehow know that? Is that why I ate grapefruit for a month?

I'm twenty-three, and sitting around with some girlfriends. The topic turns to eating disorders, and we all say we haven't had one, not exactly. I tell them about my grapefruit fast, though I can't bring myself to mention my failed attempt at bulimia. Each of them has a similar story. We talk about how much we have hated our bodies, how much we still do. I leave shocked and appalled that these beautiful, smart women can feel this way about themselves. I don't necessarily include myself in that group.

I'm twenty-five and at my writers' group. "Again with the thighs," one of the guys in the group says when they're discussing an essay I wrote on a 150-mile bike ride I did from Quincy, Massachusetts, to the end of Cape Cod.

"What?" I ask, not understanding.

"You've written here about how the thighs that you always thought of as too fat powered you up hills and across the Bourne Bridge," he says.

"Yea, so?" I ask.

"In every essay you've submitted, you talk about your thighs."

"Really?" I ask, thinking back to the pieces I've written recently, one on gardening, another on kayaking on my birthday. I don't remember any of them having to do with my thighs. And I don't think I care enough about my thighs to write about them. But apparently I do.

"Yup," he says, and other members of the group nod their heads in agreement. Now my body hatred has gotten so ingrained I don't even notice it.

I'm thirty-one and waiting for pictures of myself to download on my computer. They are from the sprint triathlon I completed a few days earlier. My body is hard and strong. I'm in the best shape of my life. And I'm proud of myself, prouder than I have ever been, prouder than when I completed two master's degrees in writing, got promoted, got married. I'm prouder because completing a triathlon seemed out of my reach in a way those other things never did. I surprised myself. And it was easier than I imagined, which means I trained well. I wasn't even particularly sore the next day.

Then the pictures appear on my screen.

The organizers had photographers set out at various points throughout the course. I saw them, and thought I smiled for the cameras. When I see the photos, though, I don't look confident and happy, the way I felt that day. I look—and I hate to say it—fat. In the photos of me running, my hips look wide in my tight, black shorts. My arms, too, have that familiar chubby look.

Before I even get through all the photos, I'm pissed at myself. When I look at pictures from the most physically grueling task of my life, I think I look fat? Really? If I heard one of the friends I did the race with say that, I would want to smack her. I want to smack myself.

Instead, I spend the next few weeks talking to all my girlfriends about my utterly ridiculous reaction to the photos. Just like when I was twenty, many of these women have similar stories of absurd thoughts they've had about their bodies. But this time, when I shake my head at how hard these beautiful, smart women are on themselves, I don't exclude myself from the group. I'm finally happy enough and proud enough of my body to realize something I never have before: photographs don't necessarily reflect the absolute, undeniable Truth. They can be taken at bad angles, under bad lighting, on bad hair days. And those crazy thoughts that run through my mind when I see a bad photo or look at myself under fluorescent lights? Those aren't necessarily the capital-T Truth, either. They're just lowercase-t thoughts.

I'm still thirty-one, standing in the bathroom, naked, as I blow-dry my hair in front of a large mirror. I think my tummy is a little pouchy. Then I think it is probably just bloated from too much caffeine yesterday. And in any case, I have better things to think about.

~Christine Junge

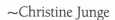

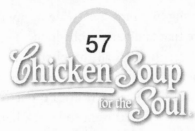

57

The After Picture

Follow your dreams, for as you dream you shall become.

~Author Unknown

Angry welts. They were the marks left on my inner thighs that brought me to tears as they burned every night.

Stretch marks. They were the ugly, deepening furrows that crept across my sides.

Sweat. It was the drops of salty water that ruined my make-up and dripped down the backs of my legs.

Clothes. I couldn't wear the pretty things I admired.

People. I read into the judging eyes behind pity smiles.

That was my "before" picture. Being overweight isn't always about being unhealthy. I tried every diet from the sensible to the extreme. The same went for my workouts. There was a time in my life when I was so desperate to lose weight that I starved myself and worked out for two hours every one of those days. The results?

I gained five pounds.

That's when I realized my body didn't react to food and exercise the way other people's seemed to. I watched friends I worked out with lose weight even as they had that extra slice of pizza I wouldn't dare to touch. Everything I ate felt like it turned to fat. I continued to beat myself up. My friends, family, and doctors were proud of my efforts, but I didn't see in terms of healthy. I saw in terms of pounds, and those pounds weren't budging an ounce.

In essence, I just wanted what every teenage girl wants: to be liked by girls and loved by boys. To me, pretty had all the advantages. They had perfect lives. They were admired.

Eventually, I resigned myself to the fate of just another "fat girl." This turned out to be one of the best decisions of my life. It was the beginning of summer, and I didn't have to worry about my weight anymore. I believed I was stuck that way forever so I might as well embrace it and live my life.

And I did.

For the first time, I focused on myself, the girl inside the "fat suit," in a way that I never had before. I stopped worrying about what other people thought of me and instead enjoyed all the good in my life. That is, all the good I had been ignoring in my quest to be thin.

I started out with little things.

I went to the mall and marched my way into what I had always called "the fat people store." Ever since I had stopped fitting into clothes at the chain stores, I was miserable and vowed to never go shopping again unless I fit into "normal clothes." I kept my promise, so this was the first time I had gone clothes shopping in over a year. The fear in me subsided after I made a few turns of the store. These weren't the bulky, baggy things I had seen overweight girls wear. They were almost stylish.

Then, I saw it. The most beautiful little, black dress I had ever seen. I automatically grabbed the largest size before I realized it was way too big. I smiled and grabbed the smallest size. At least I was a size one somewhere. With an armload of clothes, I made my way to the fitting room. Everything fit! For once, it was a matter of what I liked to wear instead of what happened to actually fit me. I walked out of that store with my head held high. Shopping was fun again.

That night, I decided to accept an invitation to go clubbing with my girlfriends. I rarely went along with them because the fact is, these girls are stunning. Going out with them is like going out with the sun. My little star was outshined every time.

But that night was different. Slowly, something was changing in me. I was smiling more. I was even laughing. For once, I was truly enjoying myself. That was when I saw him. He was tall and had these deep, dark eyes. From where I was standing, it seemed like someone had plucked Prince Charming out of a fairy tale and seated him at the table across the dance floor. Nearly every girl was staring at him. Each one would steal a glance and then move back to her clique. Even the pretty girls with the long legs and flowing, golden hair didn't have the guts to talk to him. It was about 20 minutes until closing, and I decided it was then or never.

At first, I did a little trick with my eyes. I stared intensely at the back of his head and made sure his friends saw me. Of course, they whispered to him, and he turned in my direction. He looked at me and my breath caught. He really was handsome.

Once it seemed I had "guy code" approval, I downed half a beer for dramatic effect and walked right up behind him. I could feel the judging eyes on me, but I ignored them. Instead of running away, I faked confidence and slowly ran my fingernails down his arm. Once I had his attention, I motioned him closer to me.

"Would you like to dance?"

"Sure," he grinned, and his friends cheered him on.

Frankly, I was stunned. Were those gorgeous eyes blind? I wasn't the skinny model I imagined would be on his arm.

As I took his hand and moved to the dance floor, I understood the only person standing between me and what I wanted was me.

As he danced closer, I realized he thought I was beautiful. He wasn't disgusted. He wanted to move his hands along my curves.

As the club closed down, I whispered a thank you in his ear. He said something as I left, but I didn't turn around. There would be others.

I had found confidence.

By the end of summer, I discovered romance, deepened friend-ships and finished my first novel.

With every accomplishment, I just felt good. Maybe, I even felt beautiful. The stress that had been weighing me down melted away. I was happy at long last, and with happiness came weight loss.

The more I cared about myself as a person, the more weight I lost. I was doing all the same things I had done before. I even treated myself to that slice of pizza, and the world didn't come crashing down.

I am thinner in my "after" picture, but that's not the most important change this journey has brought me. My after picture is a snapshot of a woman who allowed herself to live.

~Jennifer Azantian

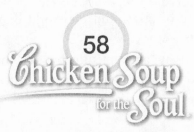

58

Just Breathe

I took a deep breath and listened to the old bray of my heart:
I am, I am, I am.
~Sylvia Plath

"Y ou have to breathe, Kyle," my nutratherapist says as I stand shaking on the scale in her office. "I can't weigh you if you're not breathing."

Still trembling, I nod and let out a small puff of air. It's my first session with her, and I've deemed her my "nutratherapist" because she's a nutritionist and a therapist rolled into one.

My heart feels like it's playing the drums, so I squeeze my eyes shut as if that will block out the sound. "Please don't tell me the number," I beg.

"I won't. I promise." She has me step down and take a seat.

I practically leap off the evil contraption and stumble over to the chair across from her desk. I watch as she writes something down on a piece of paper and folds it over so I can't see it. My weight. Oh dear God. My weight's on that piece of paper.

Those three little numbers can make or break you. Those three little numbers can make you feel beautiful or ugly. Sexy or trollish. Confident or wishing you had Harry Potter's invisibility cloak. Those three little numbers are beyond evil.

"So, tell me why you're here," she says.

I bite my lip. "I need help with my eating." I pause for a second and search for the words I need to convey my problem. "I exercise at least five times a week and count every single calorie I put into my body, but I'm still gaining weight. I don't know what else to do."

She nods and scans my chart. "You marked here that you once had an eating disorder but you got help. What made you decide you wanted to stop?"

I look down at my hands. "I dated this guy who called me fat and constantly commented on what I ate. He dumped me, obviously because he thought I was fat. So, I went on this binging and purging spree. It got out of control, and a friend convinced me to get help."

"And, you haven't purged your food since?"

I shake my head. "Absolutely not. I made a promise to my mom." I shift in my chair uncomfortably. "I should probably tell you I was also addicted to diet pills."

She nods and purses her lips together. "But, now you exercise five times a week?"

"Sometimes six," I admit.

"That's a lot, Kyle."

"Well, I have to work off my food."

She shifts in her chair, still studying me. "You count calories?"

"Yes." I fumble in my purse and whip out my iPod Touch. "I use this application on my iPod. It allows me to record everything."

"I think it's remarkable that you overcame bulimia, but I fear you've swung in a different direction. You've developed disordered eating."

My heart stops. Disordered eating?

"You've replaced your bulimic tendencies and diet pill usage with other habits that are still unhealthy: the constant need to exercise and an obsession with calorie counting."

Have I really not gotten any better? "Well, I do feel extremely guilty when I eat foods that I know I shouldn't."

She scribbles something on her notepad. "Well, who's to say you shouldn't eat them?"

I cock my head to the side and stare at her for a second, the way my dog used to when I'd talk to her. You're a nutritionist. Aren't you supposed to tell me not to eat junk food?

"Dieting doesn't work," she continues. "It just doesn't. Restricting yourself from foods you love will only backfire."

"Really?"

"How do you feel when you count calories?" she asks.

I shrug. "I don't really know. I just feel like it's something I have to do."

"Before we talk about nutrition, I think we should work on you. We have to get you to stop obsessing over food so much. Are you up for that?"

Am I up for that? What would my life be like if I didn't fixate on food all the time? What would it feel like to stop judging myself? To stop cringing every time I look in the mirror?

"The key is to eat when you're hungry and stop when you've had enough."

"That's my problem; I always want more."

She processes this and nods. "That's because you're constantly restricting yourself. Once you realize you're allowed to eat whatever you desire as long as you're hungry, the need to overindulge will subside."

Eat what I want as long as I'm hungry? Sounds crazy, but I'll try anything at this point.

She folds me into her arms and gives me a big hug. "It is criminal that someone as lovely and wonderful as you is so unhappy with herself."

I suddenly want to cry, not from sadness, but because I'm about to take a journey of self-recovery. She's right. I do have to breathe. And, I plan to start right now.

~Kyle Therese Cranston

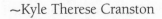

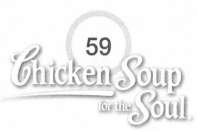

59

Photographic Evidence

Always be a first-rate version of yourself,
instead of a second-rate version of somebody else.
~Judy Garland

Photos can be powerful. Most people can probably relate to seeing a photo of themselves they hated. The absolute worst are those photos that make us look fat. I have one particular fat photo of myself that I've kept around for a laugh, but it wasn't funny the first time I saw it. I was in college and, sure enough, I'd gained "the freshman fifteen." Only in my case it was probably a bit more than that. The photo proved it. Thus began my yo-yo dieting cycle. I was terribly unhealthy. I'd skip meals or only eat salad until I went insane, then I'd have three desserts for dinner in the school cafeteria. I managed to get my weight down enough to return my borrowed clothes, but I continued doing the yo-yo thing through my senior year.

In spring of that year, I met the man who would become my husband: Chris. My weight was pretty good due to my hectic senior schedule, although I still worried about my looks. Chris, on the other hand, didn't seem to see it. In fact, after a few weeks of dating, he insisted on taking my portrait. He was quite the photographer, so he took more than just a shot or two to show me off. He took a whole roll of film — 36 pictures of me surrounded by spring blossoms in his parents' backyard. Clearly, Chris thought I was beautiful. I'd never been too sure about that.

They turned out to be powerful photos. After we'd tossed the ones with my eyes closed and with funny expressions on my face, there were some pictures of a beautiful young woman: me! While I didn't connect the dots at the time, I'm sure that those images are what led to the healthiest decision I've ever made: no more diets! I made a vow after graduating from college that I'd never "diet" again. I would focus on trying to make healthy choices without denying myself. If I wanted a piece of chocolate, I could have one—no guilt allowed! I also started to exercise more, and gradually I thought of myself as beautiful, just like Chris did, just like those photos proved.

All of this was a long time ago, but I've had cause to think about it recently. You see, Chris and I have two beautiful teenage daughters, and the older one has struggled with her weight for a long time. At the start of her junior year in high school, she was 5'8" and 180 pounds. Sadly, she felt fat. But she had an hourglass figure and a lovely face. So I encouraged her to enter a contest for plus-sized models. We had so much fun dressing up and taking her pictures! Like my first photo session with Chris, we took way more photos than we'd ever need. And it worked: just like when I saw those spring photos of me, my daughter was amazed at the photos we took of her. She was more than just beautiful—she was stunning! She didn't look fat at all. With the right clothes and the right light she looked like a movie star.

As it turned out, she didn't win the modeling contest because our faxed form didn't go through. But something even better happened. She had photographic evidence that she was a beautiful girl. With that proof, she didn't have to diet any more. Without the guilt and the shame, she didn't feel as hungry as she used to. Lo and behold, at her next doctor's visit, she had lost almost 15 pounds!

I now know that using a "fat photo" as motivation is the wrong way to go about it. To successfully lose weight you have to love yourself, just the way you are. So, use the best, most flattering picture of yourself as your motivation. After all, everybody knows a photo is worth a thousand words. But I now know that, sometimes, it can be worth a thousand calories, too.

~Annie Kuhn

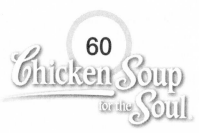

Success by Failure

Even if I don't reach all my goals, I've gone higher than I would have if I hadn't set any.

~Danielle Fotopoulis

had failed again. It was the day of the big marathon. I had resolved three years ago to train for the half-marathon event and take home a medal. There I sat, in front of my TV, while I watched others cross the finish line. It was just the latest in a long string of failures. I had never met a single weight loss or fitness goal that I had set in the last three years. I was majoring in the art of failing.

We are a family of explorers and often plan active, adventurous vacations. It seemed that on every vacation I was the one who couldn't go the distance. I had sat on massive stone steps, halfway up ancient Mayan pyramids while my family explored the antiquity and the views from the top. I had almost made it to the Great Gallery, a rare and ancient display of Indian art work painted on the side of Horseshoe Canyon in Utah. Perhaps the most humiliating failure was sitting on a mountainside in Arkansas as an old man, carrying an umbrella to shield himself from the sun, practically skipped past me on his way to the summit. He nodded to me. "Nice day for a walk," he smiled. Yeah. Sure.

Each time I urged my family, "Go on without me. Bring me lots of pictures and videos. I'll be fine just sitting here taking in the view." I lied.

Sick of being left behind, I resolved that it would never happen again. Sure I was in my 50s, overweight and obviously out of shape, but if an old man with an umbrella could skip to the top of a mountain, surely there was still hope for me. I always spent weeks of walking to prepare for our active vacations. If I hadn't, I would probably have waited in an air-conditioned car while my family went on exciting adventures without me. I had lost weight, the same weight, many times. I just always seemed to fail to get where I needed to be.

But this time I would do something different. I was going to train to walk a half marathon. Surely I would lose weight and get in shape if I could complete over 12 miles in four hours. Besides, this would be training. Training sounded cooler than diet and exercise. I was revved up and ready to go. I bought the appropriate gear, checked out what type of drinks would be handed out at the marathon and stocked up on them. I had a plan! Now two years later, there I sat, watching thousands of people of all ages succeed where I had failed.

I walked out onto the deck, frustrated with myself, sat down and held myself a pity party. I was a master at the art of pity parties, having a great deal of experience in throwing them. "I bet the old man with the umbrella runs marathons," I said to two robins on the fence. Having observed their plump bellies, I was sure they were allies.

I closed my eyes and reflected on the failures of the last three years. It was much too depressing to go back any further than that. What was my problem? Where was I going wrong? I stopped and considered each failure, one by one. I made some very interesting discoveries.

I had failed to climb to the top of that Mayan pyramid, but I did climb it and stood on those ancient stones. I failed to climb to the summit of the mountain in Arkansas, but I almost did and I had a wonderful view of the countryside and the Arkansas River. I failed to see the Great Gallery in Horseshoe Canyon but I did hike almost two miles down a steep canyon trail, three more miles through a sandy wash to see the other galleries, and then hiked two miles back up the canyon wall. I may not have gone the distance, but I didn't sit in the car either. "I have some great stories!" I shouted to the robins, who promptly vacated the fence.

I had failed to meet a single weight loss goal and yet I had lost

43 pounds. I couldn't walk 12 miles in four hours, but I could walk 12 miles. Shoot, I was even starting to do a little running.

All my failures were sounding suspiciously like a success story. Feeling much better about myself, I sat back and closed my eyes again. This time I was giving thanks. I was thankful that I had been given the spirit of failure because failure meant that I was trying, that I didn't give up, I didn't quit. I decided that at the rate I was failing, I would be crossing that finish line next year.

~Debbie Acklin

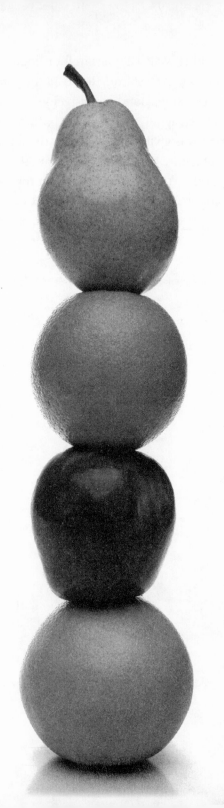

Chapter 7

Shaping the New You

Having a Partner

I will take inventory of who I am and what I want.
I will set my goals high and let nothing stop me from reaching them.

~Richard Simmons, The Book of Hope

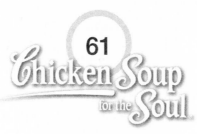

Moving

I have two doctors, my left leg and my right.
~G.M. Trevelyan

"That's it," my husband Paul announced when I walked into the kitchen after work one November evening. "I'm retiring in April."

I grabbed a bag of leftover Halloween candy and ripped it open. Water boiling for spaghetti sputtered on the stove. "Bad day?" I asked and studied his face.

"No, it's time for us to stop working and start living." Paul smiled and shrugged. "We don't know how much time we have left."

"So you want to put the house on the market and move to our place in Florida?" We had purchased a small three-bedroom home there two years earlier and used it for vacations. Eventually, we planned to relocate and retire, but I was fifty-eight and Paul was fifty-nine. I finished a handful of candy corn and shoved a whole fun-sized chocolate bar into my mouth. I reached for another.

"I'm serious," he said. "We need to do this."

And I needed to get control of my weight. When I stepped onto the scale the following morning, the number was even higher than the day before. As I dressed, I realized I felt like I was holding my breath all day to fit into my clothes. Going up to the next size loomed in the near future. Move to Florida, the land of the sun, sea, shorts and bathing suits? I didn't want to meet new people when I looked like this. My heart pounded in my chest.

But by lunchtime, I'd forgotten all about wanting to lose weight.

The roast beef dinner the cafeteria offered tempted my growling stomach, and I couldn't resist. The candy bowl threatened that evening. Finally, I just gorged myself on all the chocolate to get it out of the house. When I weighed myself the next week, the damage showed. I started taking walks on my days off, but Christmas was coming. My co-workers were bringing cookies to work. I was going to parties with so many goodies to taste. At best, I managed to keep my weight stable. I knew I shouldn't be eating this way. I was taking medication for high cholesterol. Now, my blood pressure was edging up too. Instead of moving to Florida, I was heading for the hospital.

After a few weeks of trying to lose weight on my own, I realized it wasn't working. I needed an outside authority to keep me accountable. On New Year's, I realized "that's it." Going to Florida was a chance at a fresh start, and I wanted to do it with a fit body. I decided to join a group that would provide advice and support to help me meet my goal. My friend Adele joined with me. Together, we learned the information needed to look at our eating habits. I finally saw what I was doing wrong. I went through my cabinets and pulled out all the items I would no longer eat and donated them to the local food pantry. I bought whole wheat noodles, brown rice, and seltzer to replace the spaghetti, white rice, and soda I'd removed. My biggest mistake had been drinking fruit juice with every meal. I thought I was doing something healthy and not looking at the mounting calorie count. With all these changes, I lost five pounds the first week. I could breathe in my clothes again.

Each Friday after weighing in and attending a meeting filled with tips and encouragement, Adele and I shopped at the Farmer's Market for fruit and vegetables. We joked and laughed about the advice we'd heard to encourage each other to keep going. Adele reached her goal quickly; she had less to lose. I continued walking and gradually increased my distance from one to three miles. The pounds dropped off slow and steady. One day at work, a co-worker trailing me to a meeting said, "Elaine, it's time for a new pair of pants. You've got no butt left." I had dropped two sizes and my clothing was extremely loose. I found some smaller pants to wear in another closet. I didn't want to buy any new winter clothing since we were moving. Maybe the only thing I'd need in sunny Florida would be a new bathing suit.

Paul resigned from his job in April as planned. With all the changes I'd made in our eating habits, he'd lost weight too. We started painting the house in preparation for putting it on the market. In a couple of strokes of good luck, our house sold to the first couple who called, and I received permission to work remotely from Florida since I wasn't quite ready to retire.

As I weighed in at my final doctor's appointment before the move, the nurse said, "You look great." Turned out, I was only one pound over my ideal weight.

I smiled and then beamed when the doctor told me, "Your cholesterol numbers are perfect." Not only had I lost weight, but I had achieved another goal, becoming medication-free. To celebrate, I went shopping for a size-8 summer wardrobe. That week at my last group meeting, I announced my success and hugged the group leader. "I'm so proud of you," she said. Adele echoed her sentiments, telling me I had done an amazing job.

As Paul and I packed our house for the move, I placed my large-sized clothing in a huge donation bag. "That much less to move," Paul said happily, thinking of all the boxes stacked in the garage.

We moved to Florida two years ago. We continue to care about what we eat and keep it healthy. It doesn't feel like a diet. I have dessert every day, sugar-free pudding made with fat-free milk or 100-calorie-pack cookies. Sometimes, I snack on mini-dill pickles, only five calories each. My walks have increased to five miles, and I do them most days of the week. My husband and I are known in our neighborhood as the "active" couple. And early retirement? It's everything it's cracked up to be. The best secret we've learned: just keep moving!

~Elaine Togneri

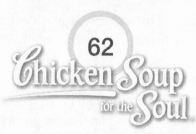

62

Partners in Craving

Food is our common ground, a universal experience.
~James Beard

I n the early days of our low-carb diet, my husband and I sat on the couch, and as if we were reading romantic love poems to each other, we recited how many carbohydrates our favorite foods had. For Valentine's Day, we had purchased pocket-sized editions of *Dr. Atkins' Carbohydrate Gram Counters* for each other instead of candy, so that we could remain loyal to each other and to the lifestyle, and not get fat again.

"Two tablespoons of cream cheese with chives and onions have only two net carbs," I said, "and they also have two grams of protein."

"That's a good one," my husband replied, "but what are we going to do? Lick it off our fingers?"

"We can have it on celery!" I said, with false enthusiasm.

We went back to our side-by-side net carb browsing and dreaming.

"Pesto sauce!" my husband said, "There are only 1.2 net carbs in two tablespoons of pesto sauce, and it has 5.6 grams of protein!" I knew his mind was where mine was, inhaling the memories of Pasta Pesto from our favorite Italian restaurant, a dish that went perfectly with their garlic bread. We hadn't been to that restaurant for many months because there were too many temptations, even though both of us admitted to dreaming about lapping up the last few drops of pesto sauce with a wedge of garlic bread.

"We can't put pesto sauce on celery," I sulked.

"Yeah, but we can put it on a steak!" my husband, the barbecue maven, said.

"That actually sounds good," I said. "But I need it on something that crunches. Like focaccia or Italian bread."

Having seen success losing weight on this diet, neither of us wanted to spoil a good thing. My husband had lost 30 pounds and was nearing his perfect weight. I had lost 60 pounds, and I now weighed less than my husband for the first time in 20 years, since before my first pregnancy. I had about 25 pounds to go to reach my ideal weight.

But nonetheless, we have our cravings.

Some couples discuss politics, the effect of El Niño, or their children. When my husband and I are relaxing, we talk about the foods we would eat if they were good for us and we did not have the tendency to gain weight. We often discuss Dairy Queen hot fudge sundaes, the smell of homemade bread baking in the oven, apple pie à la mode, and potato chips. We also discuss hot pretzels, baked potatoes with gobs of butter and sour cream, and eating Thanksgiving stuffing as a main course. But mostly, we discuss things that crunch.

My husband has even begun cooking things on the grill a bit too long so that they are charred. "You cooked the steak too long," I say.

"Yeah, but it crunches!" he replies.

~Felice Prager

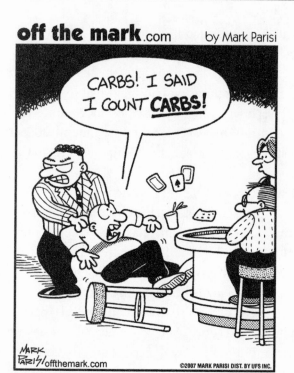

Reprinted by permission of Off the Mark
and Mark Parisi ©2007

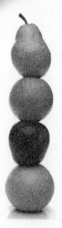

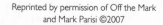

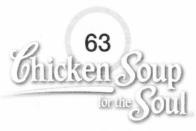

63

Vanquishing Voldemort

Determination can change your mind.
Determination can change your heart.
Determination can change your life altogether.
~Sri Chinmoy

Some are born fat and some achieve fatness. I was one of the former... my mum tells me when she laid eyes on me for the first time she was thrilled at how pink and healthy (read fat) I was. What I'd give to have been born a thin scraggly baby! My fight with fat began early. I was not even a teenager when my mum handed me a skipping rope and sat down to count my hundred jumps every day. I spent my teens picking at samosas, avoiding butter, counting calories and then bingeing helplessly.

Out of college, I found a job in Mumbai and left home. That was when my troubles began. Hostel food, no time to exercise, no time for proper meals, and the enemy returned with a whoop. Soon I was well and truly fat.

The comments followed... some funny, some irritating, some rude and some downright hurtful. However, I hadn't lived with the enemy for so long without figuring out how to handle it. I was prepared. Besides, I found a friend, Suhani. Suhani and I sat back to back in the same cubicle. She was all I was and more — fat and funny, smart and witty. The barbs seemed to bounce off her chubby frame. There was no insult she couldn't handle... no dig she didn't have a repartee to… no taunt she couldn't turn around. In fact our mutual enemy "fat" became the biggest joke between us. We christened it "Voldemort"—that almost invincible enemy, ready to pounce always. We hung around together. And we ate… how we ate! Our two-member chub club flourished.

One day, at work, I turned around to tell Suhani a particularly funny "fat" quote. To my utter shock I found her slouching on her chair. Her hands and feet stuck out at a weird angle. My heart skipped a beat. With rising panic I shook her, then splashed water on her face to no avail. Then I called for help. She was rushed to the hospital. Suhani had suffered a stroke.

I went to see her. She looked pale and helpless. She'd lost partial vision in both eyes and would be on bed for a month. She was a mere shadow of my bubbly friend. She gave me a wan smile and with a flash of her old spirit she said, "Voldemort almost got me this time, pal." The truth of her statement hit me hard. She was right. The stroke could have cost her life, left her paralysed, or worse sent her into a coma. I gave an involuntary shiver. It could've been me, was the other thought that niggled.

Voldemort was an almost invincible enemy… almost… not completely. That became the starting point for us. Once Suhani was off the bed we started morning walks, 45 minutes every day. We ate carefully but we didn't punish our taste buds. Besides the three major meals—breakfast, lunch and dinner—we made provision for two mid-meal snacks. We knew our weaknesses and worked around them. Sprout chaats, fruit salads, bhel and chutney sandwiches became the mainstay of our diet. We kept munching material handy—crunchy cucumbers, crisp apples, wheat biscuits. Our bottles of water went with us everywhere. We treated ourselves occasionally. However, if we made pasta we loaded it with veggies, skipped the cheese sauce for the tomato sauce, if we were dying for a pizza we'd have it but restrict ourselves to one slice each. Bingeing was out.

Surprisingly, the guys at work were supportive. They did jest about the end of the chub club, but not unkindly. The results were slow in coming. For almost two months nothing seemed to change. We slogged on and we waited.

Then the miracle happened. The jeans became a tad loose first, then we needed belts... wow! Then we were carrying clothes by the loads to the tailor for altering. XXLs changed to Ls. And the people were commenting. It felt... good!

We became ambitious, joined the gym while allowing ourselves the occasional slip-up. That year we celebrated Suhani's birthday with a big bang. After all it was a new life for her and for me too.

~Tulika Singh

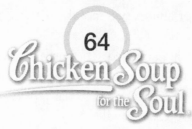

64

For Mind and Body

Exercise is good for your mind, body, and soul.
~Susie Michelle Cortright

"Want to take our walk?" My husband, home from work for his lunch break, hastily clears our sandwich plates and heads toward the door.

"Sure," I say, getting up to find my sneakers. "Bring the keys and your cell phone."

Just like that, we're off—out the garage door, walking side-by-side down the cul-de-sac. My determined, brisk strides, made prettier by my lace-adorned shoes, are no match for my husband's fast-stepping Sperry Top-Siders. We must make quite the sight, I think, looking over at my beloved, clad in his usual "business casual" attire: blue Dockers, polo shirt, and boat shoes. I pull my T-shirt down over my jeans, hoping to conceal a missing button. Sure hope we don't run into anyone we know.

A late September breeze pushes us forward, past crimson-tipped maples and yellow-leafed oaks. "Look at those gorgeous mums," I say, pointing to a home already costumed for fall. "And they have pumpkins!"

"It's a little early yet," my husband says, wisely diverting my envy. "I'll plant some flowers this weekend."

Sidestepping a lifeless white-bellied frog, we forge ahead, holding hands like teenagers. We walk a mile, past rows of colonials and stately brick Georgians. As we pass the neighborhood piano teacher's house, my worries spill out unexpectedly, like air from a popped balloon.

"Emily hasn't been practicing the piano too well," I say, wondering aloud about my parenting skills. "I just don't know if I should be sitting down next to her on the bench or letting her learn the notes on her own."

"You're doing the right thing," my husband assures me, squeezing my hand as we round another cul-de-sac. "Just be there if she needs you."

"And what about Julia?" I continue, my worries now wrapped around our younger daughter. "She burst into tears at the mere mention of choir practice."

My spouse shrugs his shoulders. "She'll end up just fine in the end—choir or no choir. Maybe she should take a break this year."

Although I'm skeptical, I feel better. The rhythmic sound of our shoes striking concrete offers steady assurance. Maybe I am on the right course. The hand in mine tells me what I already know: I have a true partner, in exercise and in life. The guy in the funny looking boat shoes will always be by my side, offering support and encouragement.

"Watch out," my husband warns as we approach a growling German Shepherd. "That thing's a beast!"

"At least there aren't any snakes today," I answer, remembering the slithering garter that surprised me by sunning himself on the sidewalk. That day, I nearly hung up my walking shoes for good.

As we circle the neighborhood, I marvel at the woodland creatures making their home in our suburban subdivision: a fluttering Monarch, a creepy, oversized cricket, a family of black squirrels. A rustling in the trees causes me to pause. A white spotted fawn looks up from his lunch of shrub leaves, eyeing us with suspicion. We are a startling sight, I suppose—this odd couple holding hands like newlyweds and circling the neighborhood each day at noon.

Despite the stares from our forest friends (and a few neighbors, waving wildly as they drive by in sports cars and SUVs), we continue to walk. A maple tree sporting the colors of fall—yellow, burnt orange and red—seems to smile upon our exercise efforts.

"Walking is really the best thing," my doctor advised at a recent physical. His eyebrows furrowed with concern for my family tree, its branches brittle with osteoporosis. "Just take a walk every day," he said. "It'll strengthen your bones."

With each measured step, I think about my mother, her once-stately 5'9" frame now a fractured 5'4". I hear echoes of my aunt's confession: "The last time I was at your house, my back hurt so badly I couldn't even find a comfortable chair."

And so, we walk—past the lake, honking geese, and yellow-tipped oaks. At the three-mile mark, I wipe my forehead, flushed yet energized from the journey.

"Want to do one more loop?" My husband looks my way, reluctant to return to his office and work routine. Perhaps walking makes him feel like I do—stronger somehow, connected down to our very bones. I wonder if we will walk forever, holding each other up through life's bumpy paths.

"Sure," I say, reaching for his hand. Crunching through the leaves, we walk side-by-side down the wooded road: a path that, for me, has made all the difference.

~Stefanie Wass

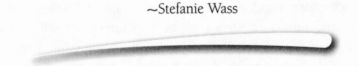

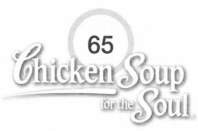

65

To Diet or Not to Diet

One's friends are that part of the human race with which one can be human.
~George Santayana

All of my friends are on a diet. Even my male friends. It's either a diet to gain weight, lose weight, redistribute weight, or maintain weight. It gets so boring. The only one who is any fun is my friend's husband who drinks light beer. That's his idea of a diet and he is going to stick to it! His paunch has retreated just a teeny bit.

We "girls" were out the other night and discovered a place that has a separate specialty menu listing how many carbs, calories and grams of protein and fat are in each serving. It also offers a low cal dessert that closely resembles a haystack sitting on chocolate syrup with a quarter teaspoon of whipped cream on top. No cherry. No nuts. We all quietly studied the diet menu. The server stopped by three times to ask us if we were ready to order. Finally, on her fourth visit she said, "How are we doing? Don't those low cal items sound tasty? Are we ready to order?"

I said, "Well, this 'we' is ready to order. I'll have the guacamole burger with fries and a chocolate milkshake. May I please have some ranch dressing on the side?"

Furiously writing and stifling a giggle, she waited for the others to order. We had asked every imaginable question about the diet menu and believe me, guacamole burgers were not on it! There was a long silence. Everyone loosened their belts a notch and said, "To heck with the diet menu!"

"I'll have chicken-fried steak with mashed potatoes and heavy on the gravy," announced the one with the least amount of weight to lose. Another spoke up, "Give me the cheese sticks, some French fries, some fried onions and a patty melt." We all giggled. She didn't really have that much weight to lose but she wanted desperately to maintain, so every time the rest of us went on a diet, she did too.

The server took our orders and we watched her gallop back to the kitchen, holding her hand over her mouth to keep from laughing out loud all the way to the chef! We actually heard a very loud, short burst of laughter from the kitchen and then muffled giggling. How rude!

We looked at each other, thumbs up and said, "Woohoo, I won't tell if you won't tell." Who were we going to tell? Each other?

Just as our feast was set before us by the giggling server, our skinniest friend walked in with her skinny husband. She stopped and asked, "How are the diets going?" We told her we were celebrating because between the three of us we had lost three pounds that week. Actually, why did we even answer her? If we'd just keep our mouths shut about dieting we wouldn't have to go through this every time someone sees us go off the wagon. We heard them order smothered pork chops and a baked potato with everything for their main course. "I bet they order dessert too," my weight-maintaining friend muttered as we made our escape. We decided to walk two blocks to the ice cream store. We called it fitness walking! And a great way to get calcium!

~Caroline Overlund-Reid

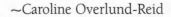

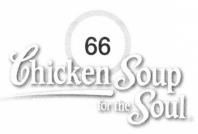

66

Ignorance Isn't Bliss

Exercise should be regarded as tribute to the heart.
~Gene Tunney

"Wow," the nurse exclaimed, staring at her lung-capacity spirometer. "You blew the top off this thing."

"I work out."

The tilt of her head and furrow in her brow said she didn't understand why I was being prepped for open-heart surgery. I exercised most of my life and ate healthy foods, including lots of fiber, vegetables and fruits. But when you inherit the big three—diabetes, high blood pressure, and heart disease—knowing the warning signs of circulatory problems is as important as all the preventative health-care I'd done in the past.

Three weeks earlier, while running at my health club, an unfamiliar pain shot down my left arm. When I slowed, the pain eased. Denial is the first human reaction but the warning sign was clear. This could be the sign of a heart problem. I'd had my diabetes under strict control for 21 years. I'd tested and controlled my blood pressure, watched my diet, and was the ideal height and weight for my age. It was easy to say, "All I need is a little rest."

A week later the same thing happened. I had no problem lifting the heavy weights, but when I ran on the track that pain reoccurred, shooting down my arm. It was time to schedule a treadmill test. Less than five minutes into the test, the doctor prepared me for an angiogram.

Four days before my 59th birthday, I had quadruple bypass surgery. My cardiologist and my surgeon were excellent and my recovery swift. When I visited my surgeon for a post-op checkup, he said, "You need to watch your cholesterol, saturated fats, diet and exercise, or I'll be doing another one of these in three to four years."

Anger rose in me, but common sense pushed it back down. My primary care physician knew my past history. My surgeon only knew what those arteries looked like when he'd performed the operation. I had to admit that before I was diagnosed with diabetes 21 years earlier, I didn't care what I ate. I didn't run or exercise like I should have.

"My cholesterol is normal, and my HDL is high," I said. "I eat a strict diabetic diet and work out four to five times a week."

He nodded, smiled, and said, "Keep it up."

As the months went by, my wife, Pam, and I made a game plan for health improvement for both of us. My ordeal had been her ordeal as well. Sitting in the hospital's waiting room wondering whether her husband would survive the operation wasn't an experience she ever wanted to go through again. Neither did I. God and I had a little talk while I lay on that gurney before the operation, and I told Him I wanted to be around for my wife on our 60th wedding anniversary. Our plan was simple. We were going to do everything we could to live a healthy life.

Pam researched foods, fats, and sodium. Sodium was the only culprit we were abusing, and we made drastic cuts. We read the labels on canned food, buying low or no sodium products whenever possible.

My wife and I have always exercised together. Each of us has a different regimen for weights and body toning, but we worked the track together encouraging each other to go an extra lap or two.

It took me five years to regain the athletic prowess I'd had before the surgery. My doctor told me to be careful with any exercise that put stress on my sternum where the ribs were pulled apart, even after it was fully healed. It took a few years to figure out what I could do and what I should avoid. So weight training came back slowly.

But cardio work, which I prefer to do on the indoor track, returned quickly. Within two months, I blew the top off that spirometer once again.

Today, I don't try to run as fast as the 20-somethings. I don't try to lift more weight than the 30-somethings. I find that doing more reps at lower weights is more beneficial to me than trying to lift heavier and heavier weights. I'm what they call an ectomorph. My tall slender body type doesn't build massive muscles and now at a healthy sixty-seven years old, enjoying my work out is more important. So when chided by the younger guys with, "Come on, bro, drop down a few more plates on that machine." I simply say, "Nope. I'm fine with this."

If my workout achieves my personal goals, and I have the desire to keep coming back, I'm doing what's right for me. I avoid that macho thing I have embedded in my psyche and use common sense.

My wife and I briskly walk uphill from our car to the athletic center—about a quarter mile. We work our own weight and limbering programs for 30 to 35 minutes, and then we hit the track together. I can obtain a great cardio workout without lapping her on the track. Instead, I stay beside her, and we talk and share our thoughts. I find the experience to be quite romantic. We'll be celebrating our 45th wedding anniversary next year and romance is still in fashion. Take good care of your health; it is worth it.

Nine years have passed since that open-heart surgery. My exercise program is as good as or better than before the bypass. I'm very well educated on all the problems associated with diabetes, high blood pressure, and heart disease. I may have inherited these conditions but I don't have to be crippled by them. Ignorance isn't bliss! Had I not exercised and known my body, I might have missed the warning signs. I might not have felt any pain, and my wife could have been a widow at age fifty-six.

I've never been back to my heart surgeon. He's the best and I owe him my life. My cardiologist and my primary care physician are a different story. They keep testing how I'm doing with stress tests and physical exams. Could I need open-heart surgery again? Yes, with insulin-dependent diabetes the long-term effects keep adding up. But if I keep doing everything I can do, and medical science does everything it can do, an enjoyable life lies ahead of me.

My wife and I count our blessings every day. Retirement isn't a death sentence. But if we hadn't taken care of ourselves in our 40s and 50s, we might never have reached our 60s with the energy and joy of living we feel. As I finish this writing, it's 11 o'clock on a Wednesday. I only have 45 minutes to clean off my desk and head out to the gym. The sun's shining. The wind is a bit brisk. Pam and I are going to pick up our son on his lunch break and work out with him too.

~Bill Wetterman

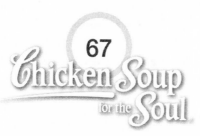

67

My Friends Are Losers

The only competition of a wise man is with himself.
~Washington Allston

An e-mail message was sent out to see if there was any interest in a faculty-wide weight loss competition. I deleted it. I had many reasons for not wanting to participate: too time-consuming, too costly, too personal. My weight was not something I planned to discuss with my co-workers. It just didn't feel right.

After the first e-mail message, there was another. Several teachers had signed up but the group leader was recruiting more. I heard co-workers chatting about weight loss goals and tips. It was the main topic of discussion in the English and History departments.

"Have you signed up for Prince George biggest losers?" a co-worker asked.

"No, I haven't. I don't really have the time for that right now," I lied.

Really? The time? The more I thought about it, the more ridiculous it sounded. I was declining the opportunity to improve my health because I didn't have time for a weekly weigh-in and a brief meeting. I was starting to re-think my decision.

My friend, Anna, and I were walking to the faculty lounge to get some coffee when she told me she had decided to join the group.

"Have you thought about it?" she asked. "We could be weigh-in buddies. It might be fun."

Talking with Anna made me realize that I had not seen all of the potential benefits of joining. At the end of our discussion, I returned to my work area and fired off an e-mail to the gym teacher, our weight loss group leader. After all, what did I have to lose? Well, about 25 pounds to be exact.

"Ms. Gilbert, please add me to the list of participants. I will be at the first meeting next Friday."

Ms. Gilbert made folders for all of the participants that contained charts for weight and measurements and some tips for healthy eating and exercise. At our first meeting, we recorded our initial weight and discussed the rules of the program. We would weigh in each Friday morning with our partners. We would pay two dollars per week for 16 weeks. There would be a weekly cash prize awarded as well as two grand prizes, one for the most pounds lost and one for most inches.

I didn't make too many immediate changes to my diet. I just quit eating late night snacks, switched to diet sodas, and drank black coffee.

At the first official weigh-in, I recorded a loss of eight and a half pounds. I was quite pleased. I was even happier when I found out that was the week's biggest loss and I was taking home 25 dollars.

As the weeks went by, I continued making small changes to my diet. I drank more water, ate more salads, decreased the size of my dinner, and avoided second helpings. I wasn't losing weight quickly; but I also didn't feel like I was suffering. That was important to me. If I gave up too much too quickly, I was afraid I might become frustrated and quit.

A few weeks into the program, co-workers began commenting on my appearance.

"Those pants are sagging off your behind," one lady said. "It's time for you to go shopping for some new clothes."

I thanked her graciously for the compliment. It felt great to have my hard work noticed by someone other than immediate family. I was encouraged by the positive comments and I continued down my path of exercise and better eating.

About a month later, I won the weekly competition a second time. At that point, I had lost a total of 12 pounds.

I was steadily losing weight and I could feel myself becoming more confident. My tummy wasn't protruding and my double chin was retreating.

And in addition to my personal loss, I was also enjoying being a cheerleader for co-workers. We congratulated one another in the hallways and shared our success stories. I felt connected to others as we worked towards a common goal.

The middle of December finally arrived and it was time for our last weigh-in. I didn't lose anything that week—not a single pound. I also didn't gain. But I knew that no loss would hurt my chance of an overall win.

I was not the school's biggest loser. I lost a total of 19 pounds but there were three other people who lost more. I was happy for them. Everything about the experience had been positive and I was really glad I had participated.

When school opened after winter break, an e-mail was sent out to see if there was any interest in a second weight loss competition. I didn't waste any time making that decision. After all, what did I have to lose? Honestly, about 10 more pounds. And what did I stand to gain? More self-confidence, friendships, and improved health.

I signed up right away.

~Melissa Face

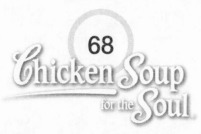

My Husband
Is on a Diet

I love being married. It's so great to find that one special person
you want to annoy for the rest of your life.
~Rita Rudner

"I hate myself," my husband, Bob, said, trying on a new pair of shorts. "I ate those curly fries last night." He turned this way and that in front of the mirror. "Do these make me look hippy?"

"No Bob. Nothing makes you look hippy. You're thin, okay? You've been thin all your rotten life. Do you understand what I am saying?"

He didn't get my tone. The tone that means I intensely resent his ability to lose weight by switching from thick-sliced bacon to the regular kind.

"Besides," I said. "What's wrong with eating curly fries once in a while?"

"Helloooo?" He looked at me incredulously. "Potatoes? Water retention?" He threw his hands up in the air. "Don't get me started."

Then he got on the scale. "Oy, I'm still plateauing."

He scanned his body in the mirror. "I have my mother's thighs." Then he pinched his tiny waist. "If you can pinch an inch, it's time to cinch." He tightened his belt one notch. "This way I'll stay motivated."

Living with a dieter is a pain.

Living with a successful dieter is hell.

Now you know I want my husband to be healthy. I just wouldn't mind if it entailed, at the very least, a teeny minor struggle to do it.

He just had a physical. I was happy he was getting his cholesterol tested because he eats so much crap I figured he needed a wake-up call. His cholesterol number came back a terrific 156. You can blame it on genetics. You can blame it on whether or not you were breast-fed. You can blame it on solar storms or some 666 devil thing. I don't care what you blame it on. I blame it on Bob.

Last night, he screamed from the bathtub. "I've got it!"

I called out from the den. "Geez, Bob. I'd hate to think what you mean by that."

"It's my metabolism." He was reading a women's magazine and eating his after-dinner jelly sandwich. "With all this starvation and yo-yo dieting, it's come to a halt."

I could hear him getting out of the tub and slamming the magazine on the floor. He shouted, "If you're not reed-thin like these models, then you're made to feel like a glutton."

"You are a glutton."

Do I sound resentful? You bet I am. His favorite dining companion? Oscar Mayer. My husband thinks peanut butter is a seasoning.

A major part of this problem is that Bob, like many males, wouldn't gain weight on an IV of Wesson Oil. I just love being married to someone who programmed Papa Gino's before 911 on our speed dial.

If you're feeling sorry for Bob, I don't blame you. But try to picture what it's like living with someone who thinks burritos are a food group.

Attempting to be sympathetic with me, which is never a smart idea, he said, "I know it's not fair that I can eat whatever I want."

"Fair? Sure it is." I was starting a slow burn. "You struggle too. You want extra-cheese pizza all the time, but you deny yourself by only having it on days of the week that end with the letters d-a-y."

As of today, I will try to be nice about it. Maybe you could try too. If you see him, please say something encouraging like, "The extra weight makes you look younger." That ought to make his day, or mine!

~Saralee Perel

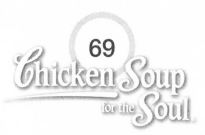

Bridge
to Life

Shoot for the moon.
Even if you miss, you'll land among the stars.
~Les Brown

I was forty-five years old and weighed 396 pounds. Getting in and out of the car was all the exercise I could manage. I walked around the grocery store leaning heavily on the shopping cart for support. How could this have happened to me?

In high school I excelled at sports. Track was my favorite. On the wall of my office the framed state medal for the 440-yard relay still held a prominent spot. What happened to the person I used to be? I wondered how long a 396-pound woman could expect to live.

I wanted to make a change. Change or die. I was embarrassed and ashamed, but I knew I had to reach out for understanding, encouragement, and support. I called one of my college friends who lived across the state. She hadn't seen me in decades.

"It doesn't matter where we've been," said Maggie. "It's where we're going."

"We?"

"I've gained weight, too," she admitted. "And although I'm not as large as you are, my health is deteriorating. It's now or never. Let's do this together."

We regularly checked in with each other. In just a few months, she reported that she'd walked a whole mile. The time it took her didn't matter. A mile is a mile.

My own progress was not so rapid. The milestones I accomplished were more on the "I made it to the first bench on the boardwalk without stopping to rest" variety.

But days and weeks turned into months, and then an entire year had passed. Maggie was able to jog two to three miles a day, and I was now fit enough to quickly walk the same distance.

"Don't they have some kind of bridge run/walk thing over by you?" she queried one day early that spring.

"The Great Columbia Crossing," I replied. "It's held on the second Sunday in October every year. It's advertised as a 10K event that traverses the Astoria-Megler Bridge. The brochure says it's a mostly flat run with a 'challenging incline' near the end."

"Challenging incline?"

"It's almost a quarter mile straight up and over the shipping channel on the Columbia River."

"Good grief," she laughed. "I guess we'll have to start training on hills."

"You can't be serious."

But she was serious. And on the second Sunday in October, after she drove eight hours to join me, I stood beside her as Maggie signed the entry form and received her T-shirt. It was a bittersweet moment. I couldn't go with her, not even to walk. Although my weight was down to 238, I had developed a painful heel spur and my physical activities were limited to the swimming pool until I could have surgery.

Maggie completed the bridge run in fine time. It was a day of celebration.

But for me, the real celebration came a year later, when I was able to complete the crossing myself, sans bone spur and another 70 pounds. My time wasn't so great, mostly due to the fact that I'd stopped at the top of the "challenging incline" to have my picture taken in the "Rocky Balboa victory salute."

I'm grinning like a Cheshire cat in that picture, but if you look closely enough, you'll also see my tears of joy.

~Jan Bono

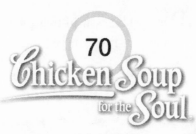

70

It Pays to Keep Walking

Afoot and light-hearted I take to the open road,
Healthy, free, the world before me,
The long brown path before me leading wherever I choose.
~Walt Whitman

My husband and I are both very creative. Dave is currently the househusband, but in his spare time he plays guitar and writes songs. I sew quilts and do freelance writing when I'm home from my full-time job. We are building our own house from the ground up. As a result of constantly being involved in our projects, we are not very sports-minded. The most activity I usually do outside is gardening, and Dave fixes our vehicles himself and runs most of the errands around town. We are involved in church activities and we play with our grandkids. But most of what we do is indoors, sitting down.

We've had quite a few medical problems and managed to rack up a lot of bills in the past for doctors and medical tests. Then in 2007 Dave had a heart attack and I was diagnosed with the muscle disorder fibromyalgia. We took a good look at making some lifestyle changes. Dave worked on the meal planning, which I benefited from as well. We both started losing weight. But we were also advised to get more exercise.

Walking. That's all we needed to do. Just walk every day. Somehow that just didn't fit in with our normal schedule, and we knew we were in for a challenge. We had already tried going to a gym, using a treadmill, etc. but nothing worked to keep us walking. Even just remembering to walk every day was a drawback for both of us.

Our latest medical issues provided new incentive to get more serious about this, so we made our usual resolution to walk more. Dave drove down to the small lake below us and walked around it nearly every day, a good half hour of exercise. He admired the scenery, took pictures of the ducks and geese, and seemed to be doing fine with this routine, for a while. But as the initial shock of having a heart attack began to wear off, daily distractions took over and Dave began to plan less time-consuming exercise. A brisk walk down to the "Y" in our dirt road and back up the other side took only 20 minutes and was up- and downhill. That seemed to work at first. But he gradually grew more forgetful and when the weather was bad, it was difficult to keep it up.

My daily walking needed to be mostly at work because by the time I got home, I was too tired to do anything. Sometimes I even had to take a nap because of my fibromyalgia. I resolved that I would get away from the desk at break times and walk for 10 minutes. Two breaks would be 20 minutes. Unfortunately, I tended to be less dedicated when it was too hot, or too cold, or raining, or snowing, or I was too achy, or I wanted or needed to do something else during my break! I knew if I walked more I would feel better and maybe not need so many naps, but I still struggled with walking every day. However, my real worry was Dave. He had a life-threatening possibility if he didn't keep up his walking. Something had to be done, so I prayed for a way to keep us both motivated to walk.

At last one day I had an idea. It seemed kind of silly at first, but I actually thought it might work so I told Dave about it. What if we paid ourselves to walk? My plan was this: we would each keep track of our walking time on the calendar, adding it up as "walking points." Whenever we reached 120 points, we would get $10 to spend or save for whatever we wanted. In addition to the money, I figured there would be a little competition, which might add to the motivation.

Since our money is always budgeted for bills and living expenses, or catching up on credit cards, we don't often have anything extra to buy things that are not necessary. Dave is always window-shopping in catalogs and online for electronic equipment to go with his music playing or song recording. Yet he almost never has the opportunity to buy any. I often want some clothes or certain books that are out of our price range.

Dave liked the idea, so we started applying it, and to our surprise, it worked! Dave soon began keeping up his 20 minutes a day. One of the first things Dave bought was a bass guitar. (Now that's incentive!) Another time he got an MP3 player. As I write this, he has saved up $155 for some unknown item he hasn't decided on yet.

The plan worked for me as well. I was now more inclined to walk at work during my break time. There was a certain pair of fancy shoes I wanted to buy, and a $50 sweater in a catalog. I found myself walking specifically to earn points to be able to get those items.

The competitive side of the plan worked as well. We found ourselves telling others that we had to go out for walks so we could earn our walking points. "Dave is way ahead of me this week," I would say. One time I kept forgetting something in the car at a large church gathering outdoors, and Dave teased me. "You're just walking back to the car so you can get more points!"

When I first thought of this idea, I also wondered how we could afford it. But as I told Dave at the time, if we kept walking we might save on medical bills. Didn't it make sense to stay healthier and not need a doctor? We had spent thousands of dollars on medical bills in the past. Why not spend it on ourselves to stay healthy?

For us, this plan has worked 18 months and counting. Sometimes I just want $10 for something special, and other times I save it up for something more expensive. And thank God, we have been healthier—what a bonus! Our doctor bills have been generally lower this past year. Could it be that the walking points plan not only kept us walking but also actually saved us money?

We may never know the answer to that, but one thing we can say for sure: it definitely pays to keep walking!

~Laurie Penner

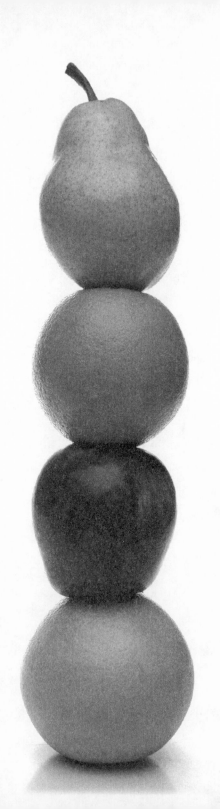

Chapter 8

Shaping
the
New
You

Telling Myself the Truth

The most important promises for me to keep are the ones I made to myself.

~*Richard Simmons*, The Book of Hope

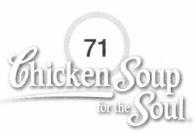

Lying to Myself

The body never lies.
~Martha Graham

"There's no way she's going to actually read them," I assured my friend Renée. "She'll never know." We stifled our giggles in the back of the seventh-grade science classroom, where our teacher had just given us a nutrition assignment: write down everything you eat for one whole week. I knew Mrs. Beacham would merely check them off but not read them.

One week later, we compared our lists. We read the more unusual "meals" on each others' lists: a wheel of cheese, a meatloaf milkshake, and an entry for which I took top prize—seven Star Wars figures. "Ooh, you forgot something," Renée laughed, penciling in the words "with salt." "No one would eat those things plain."

Mrs. Beacham never questioned us about our strange eating habits or called social services to report what our parents were serving us. It was the first time I lied about what I had eaten.

As an adult with a weight problem, I became a veteran food journaler. I watched talk shows on weight loss, clipped columns on healthy eating, and highlighted numerous diet books. I knew that keeping a food journal was an important tool for losing weight. I just wasn't sure why.

So I kept diet journal after diet journal, filling one blank book and moving on to the next as the years went by and the pounds piled on. It was a cinch, especially because I didn't write down every single thing I ate. It wasn't necessary, I told myself, as long as the main foods were there. I would scrawl "salad and iced tea" for lunch, neglecting to mention that the salad came with a basket of breadsticks dripping in butter, or that I "tasted" my co-worker's pound cake that she didn't want to finish. "Those are negligible calories," I told myself, shutting the book.

Almost anything could be "negligible calories" in those days. Food tasted while cooking for my family? Negligible. Samples at the grocery store? Negligible. From wedding cake to cocktails to late night potato chips, you guessed it: negligible, negligible, negligible. It's a wonder I wrote anything down at all, but I was insistent on tracking my main meals of the day. The trouble was, I was eating even more outside of mealtimes than I was at the meals themselves. I just didn't know it yet.

One day a co-worker gave chocolates to all of us. Sheila, whose desk was next to mine, popped hers into her mouth at the same time as me, while we both rolled our eyes and made appreciative noises. "Oh, wait," Sheila remembered. "Gotta write that down." She scrambled for a book in her bag. "Food journal," she explained, and made a notation.

"You're writing down that chocolate?" I asked.

"Sure," she said. "I keep track of everything I eat. Each one of those little things has thirty calories."

"Thirty calories surely won't make that big a difference," I said. "It's... negligible."

"Oh, 30 calories might be negligible, but over the whole day it can add up. Thirty calories here, 50 calories there... before you know it, you've eaten a whole extra meal's worth in a day. By the end of the week that can mean a whole extra pound. If I write it down, I know to be careful the rest of the day. No more extra treats. But one's okay," she said. "You need some small perks. Otherwise I wouldn't have lost these last 10 pounds."

Ten pounds? That's what I'd gained since my last weigh-in at the doctor. Here was someone whose scale was actually going in the opposite direction from mine. Was she more successful than me because she was writing down every single thing that she ate? It just seemed like such a waste of time. I kept a food journal too; I just wasn't a slave to it.

I decided to give it one week. I would keep my food journal Sheila's way: writing down every single thing that passed my lips. I would even count the calories.

By the end of day one I was manic. How many calories are in one handful of peanuts anyway? I looked online and rounded the number up to be on the safe side. All of my nibbles here and there were impossible to calculate. What's one-fourth of a candy bar? Half a cola? Does anyone know how many doughnut holes make a dough-nut? I was up to my eyeballs in measurements and fractions, and worst of all: calorie counting.

The next day I caught Sheila by the elevator. "I wanted to ask you some questions about your food journal," I said. I told her my difficulty keeping track for just one day. "How do you even have time to calculate all these nibbles throughout the day?"

"Oh, that's easy," she answered. "I had just as hard a time as you. It was a headache! That's when I discovered there was a much easier way. I quit eating that stuff."

"Really?" I asked. "But that chocolate..."

"Like I said, that was a treat. I write down everything I eat, and I do it meticulously, but it's a whole lot simpler if I stick to meals and the healthy snacks I bring from home. Sometimes I even write it all down in the morning when I pack it, so I'm obliged to eat only what I planned."

"Wow," I marveled. "That's really smart. Thanks, Sheila."

"Sure thing," she said. "But I thought you were the food journal expert. You've carried one around as long as I've worked here."

"That's true," I confessed, "but I wasn't always truthful in it. I hadn't been writing down what I really ate."

"You lied to your food journal?" she laughed. "That's hilarious. Who did you think was going to read it?"

I laughed too, but I felt strange. When I got home that night I pulled out my old food journals and really looked at them. While

I knew I had cut corners, it wasn't until Sheila had said the word that I saw them for what they really were: lies. I had lied to my food journal. And what was worse, as Sheila had pointed out, no one else was going to see them. That means I was lying to myself.

Incredulously, I scanned through pages and pages of "salad" and "sandwich," knowing that the salads were drenched in dressing, the sandwiches were sometimes a foot long, and the snacks were missing altogether. I had been writing fiction. My food journal was as much a lie as if it said "seven Star Wars figures, with salt."

I started writing down everything I ate, even when it was hard to calculate, and even when it seemed "negligible." And like Sheila, I eventually found myself passing on snacks just to make my calculations simpler. My new accountability led to a steady weight loss that I owe completely to my food journal—my new and improved, one hundred percent factual food journal.

Now I look back in disbelief at the heavier me who wrote a fake food journal. Today, if I were to write down "seven Star Wars figures," you can bet your life that I would have had action figures for lunch. No salt, though: sodium can make you bloated.

~Elizabeth Kelly

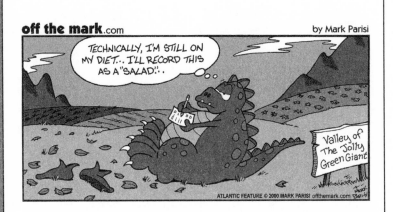

off the mark.com   by Mark Parisi

TECHNICALLY, I'M STILL ON MY DIET... I'LL RECORD THIS AS A "SALAD"...

Valley of The Jolly Green Giant

ATLANTIC FEATURE © 2000 MARK PARISI! offthemark.com

Reprinted by permission of Off the Mark
and Mark Parisi ©2000

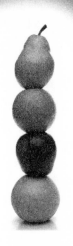

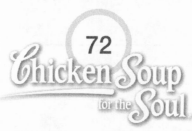

72

A Weighty Revelation

To feel "fit as a fiddle," you must tone down your middle.
~Anonymous

When Bob and I got married 39 years ago, he weighed a good 50 pounds more than I did. I'd been self-conscious for years, being one of the tallest in my class at 5'9"... taller than many of the boys in my high school. That was a hard insecurity to shake. To realize that Bob was "bigger" than I was weight-wise was a welcome boost for my self-esteem.

I enthusiastically welcomed my added pounds and beach-ball contours when I became pregnant with our children, Jennifer and Wade, but managed to stay active enough afterwards to drop those extra pounds and reclaim my original shape. Now that decades have passed, my metabolism has crashed, and our kids have grown and left us with an empty nest; my waistline and the numbers on our scales seem to be growing uncontrollably.

I used to try dieting, but Jen and Wade told me to eat because I was too grouchy. I've half-heartedly tried to eat more healthily, yet realize eating healthy meals isn't enough. I still find myself sneaking the sweets I crave—and I know my body deserves better. Those calories are not only fattening, they're dangerous to my health. My brain knows this, but my mouth and taste buds betray me when I least expect it... and I'm disappointed in my lack of self-discipline.

I used to run for exercise until my joints gave out. I powerwalk and work out at the gym now, but since my hips and waist stubbornly stay the same, perhaps that's not enough.

Some try to tell us not to worry about the actual size of clothes we wear... what matters is for our clothing to fit well. Reluctantly, I recently followed that advice and swallowed my pride as I purchased a size of jeans I swore I'd never buy. I needed some "well-fitting" jeans to take on a weekend trip with Bob. Yes, the size was hard to accept, but they were made with "stretch" denim, and the labels said they would make my tummy "seem slimmer." That dulled my ego's pain a little.

I hoped these were the right choice of jeans, because I wanted to look and feel my best on this romantic getaway to a picturesque southern New Mexico lodge Bob had heard about. The inn was lovely and the room we stayed in was quaint, albeit very tiny. That meant the little dresser only had a couple of small drawers and there was no closet.

Because of the lack of space, I just folded my new jeans and placed them on a shelf. I planned to wear them the next morning on a scenic drive and hike which Bob was anxious to share with me.

When I came out of the diminutive bathroom, drying off from my shower, I found Bob standing in front of the mirror with a puzzled look... staring at the pants he'd just zipped up. "What's wrong with these jeans? The pockets are in the wrong place and the legs don't feel right."

"No!" I gasped in horror. "I laid your jeans out on the chair. You're wearing mine!" Bob just laughed, but I was devastated. After 39 years of marriage, Bob put on the wrong pants and they fit him.

I tried to tell myself the reason they fit was because of the stretchy denim, but knew in my breaking heart that I could no longer deny it. I'm as big around the middle now as Bob is. I don't know how much Bob actually weighs, but even though he still weighs more than I do, I'm sad to admit that my body's shape has morphed into his twin.

This wrong-pants revelation has given me a new determination and focus to get my act together.

I was blessed with good health and a slim body in my youth, and I became lazy. I'm grateful to be older now, but with that gift, I need to take more responsibility. I know I can do this. I deserve it.

I can no longer be lazy and just eat whatever… whenever, because I want to live a long, happy life with my husband and dear family. Sweets and fatty foods must be cut out, and as long as I'm physically able, I want to push myself harder at the gym and take more frequent walks. I have no desire to be the size I was at our wedding, but I do need to take better care of myself.

If I can firm up and slim down at least enough that Bob can never wear my jeans again, I'll be thrilled… yet I know that shouldn't be my only reason. They say what's really important is to be healthy, but my new determination to try harder makes me feel better about myself. That's important too. Bob has always loved and supported me, but even after being married 39 years, I realize some of my insecurities still linger. By no longer being lazy and taking better care of myself, I will grow as a person. That's much better than growing around my middle! Bob may have picked the wrong pants, but I know now more than ever that he picked the right woman.

~Lynne S. Albers

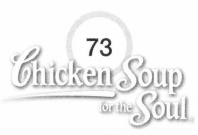

73

A Bag of Potatoes

To lengthen thy Life, lessen thy meals.
~Benjamin Franklin

I squinted at the woman in the photo taken at my aunt's birthday party. "Who is that fat lady sitting next to Uncle John?" I asked, "I don't recognize her."

My aunt hesitated and then answered, "It's you."

I was shocked. The fat lady I didn't recognize was me!

I looked at the photo again. It really was me. It wasn't the "me" I thought I was—it was the "real" me.

I was fat. I was 50 pounds overweight. I'd gained it all in the past two years. I was putting on 25 pounds a year and at this rate I wouldn't live long because diabetes and heart trouble run in my family.

I went to a doctor expecting him to give me a medical reason for my rapid weight gain.

"You're two pounds away from being obese because you eat too much and you don't exercise. Lose weight or die," he said.

Obese? Die?

I'd been living in denial for two years. I'd noticed I was buying clothing that was extra large when I used to be a size 10. It was harder to bend over, tie my shoes, climb stairs and trim my toenails. I told myself I was just getting old. I never told myself I was getting fat.

It was easier to blame it on my age. After all, no one can help getting old.

If my problems were because I was fat, that made me, and me alone, responsible.

It wasn't about food. It wasn't about hunger. It was about loneliness, boredom and depression.

I was lonely. I was divorced and my children had grown up and left home. I was used to taking care of other people. Now that I was alone, I wasn't motivated to take care of myself.

I'd been using excuses for not dieting or exercising: If I had a man in my life, I'd have a reason to lose weight. If I had a social life, I'd care about how I looked. If my children visited me more often, I'd get into shape so I could go places with them. If I had a friend to diet and exercise with... If...

Now I realized that I had to take care of myself because I was worth it. That had to be a good enough reason.

When I was at the market I saw large bags of potatoes. Each bag held 10 pounds of potatoes. I felt like a bag of potatoes, heavy and lumpy and bumpy, dull and uninteresting.

I stacked up five bags to represent 50 pounds.

I was carrying around the equivalent of these five bags of potatoes every day.

I bought one bag of potatoes and took it home. It represented one-fifth of my excess weight. I carried the bag of potatoes with me constantly, up stairs, down stairs, every step I took. When I sat down to watch TV, the sack of potatoes sat on my lap like a baby.

I ate smaller portions of food and used a saucer instead of a plate. I ate four small meals a day and nothing but fruit or water after sunset.

I put the bathroom scale in front of the refrigerator and weighed myself every time I opened the door to get food. I found I opened it a lot less. I taped the "fat" photo of myself on the bathroom mirror to remind me how I never wanted to look again.

When I lost the first pound, I removed a potato from the bag. Each time I lost a pound I'd take out another potato. When I lost 10 pounds and the bag was empty, I bought another bag of potatoes and started over.

When people began to notice I'd lost weight I told them I was on the "Potato Diet"—I don't eat the potatoes, I carry them around!

I've lost 31 pounds so far, more than half my goal.

I can climb stairs without puffing. I can trim my toenails without looking like a contortionist.

When I started to control what I ate, I gained control over other areas of my life. I had more money because I wasn't wasting it on junk food and having pizza delivered twice a week. I was saving over $100 a month on pizza alone and put the money into a special account for a new wardrobe after I've lost 50 pounds.

My house is cleaner because I have more energy and it doesn't seem like such an effort to do housework.

I feel better about myself and I'm happier and more cheerful. I've been walking to the library and have joined a book discussion group and made some new friends.

My life has changed.

The next time I see myself in a photo, I'll say, "I know that lady! It's me!" and I'll feel proud.

~April Knight

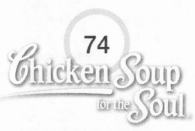

74

Cheating that Works

It is impossible for a man to be cheated by anyone but himself.
~Ralph Waldo Emerson

I only cheated on an exam once. It was in middle school and I happened to catch a glimpse of my friend's math paper and saw that her answer to a question differed greatly from mine. After a brief ethical tussle, I succumbed, erased my numbers, and then hastily scribbled in hers. Although that answer was correct, the remaining answers on my test were not. I didn't cheat again.

Until now. This time, it was a test of willpower. I'm on a special diet with foods carefully selected for balanced nutrition and caloric value. A piece of cheesecake is not an option. So here was my dilemma:

Should I...

    A. eat the cheesecake and spend the rest of the week berating myself for my lack of willpower?

    B. eat the cheesecake, pretend I didn't and then blame any weight gain on a broken bathroom scale?

    C. not eat the cheesecake, feel surly and take out my frustration on the annoyingly skinny and perky aerobics instructor at the gym?

    D. eat the cheesecake and work off the calories?

Choice D seemed like a win-win solution. Not only would I get to enjoy the cheesecake, but I'd get an exercise session. Knowing my lack of follow through, I knew that if I devoured the treat before the exercise, I'd rather wallow in my guilt than get off my duff. And then it hit me: an ingenious plan to use my cheesecake as an exercise incentive. I plated a thin slice of cheesecake and carefully walked it up the stairs and set it on my bedside table with a small fork. I donned my exercise outfit and went downstairs.

The lure of the cheesecake got stronger so I launched my plan: I would run up and down the stairs and then back up again. My reward: one small bite of cheesecake. If I wanted another, I'd have to run down and up and down and up again. Off I went. Ah, creamy vanilla goodness without guilt. I wanted another bite so I quickly sprinted through another stair-climbing run.

Admittedly, it is harder to savor the creaminess of the cheesecake when my tongue was dry from panting. I placed a bottle of water next to the cake.

Down and up and down and up again. When I trudged over to the cheesecake, my hand bypassed the plate and went for the water instead. I didn't want the darned cake anymore. I'd rather all this sweat and effort do more than offset the calories from cheesecake. I was exhausted and I'd have nothing to show for it. The scale wouldn't move; my waist wouldn't shrink. Sure the cheesecake tasted fine but just not good enough to make me run up and down the stairs one more time.

My plan worked. Now, anytime I felt tempted to indulge in a former favorite, I remembered my stairs trick.

I learned that other diet cheaters use their own cheating rules. They are surprisingly effective. Here are two:

1. The Drown It Rule: In order to eat a bite of the forbidden food, you first must drink an entire eight-ounce glass of water and wait 10 minutes. Then, you can have one bite. If you want another bite, you have to repeat the water drinking and waiting routine. This keeps the cheating to a minimum as your stomach fills with liquid and as your brain receives the fullness signal.

2. The One-Inch Rule: You can cheat and eat anything you want as long as you keep it to a one-inch piece only once a day. The extra calories from a small bite, once a day, should not affect your overall daily caloric intake by much.

Unfortunately, my husband doesn't play by the rules. He saw the half-eaten cheesecake in the bedroom and finished it while watching Discovery Channel in bed. "Hey, that's not how it's supposed to go," I said. "You can't eat a bite until you run down and up the stairs."

"Why?"

"That's the rule of cheating."

"There are no rules to cheating. Cheating breaks the rules."

"I know, but in order not to really be cheating, you just follow a new set of rules," I explained. "This one calls for you to run up and down the stairs if you want to take a bite of cheesecake."

"Who made up this rule?" he asked, scraping the plate with the side of the fork.

"I did," I replied, proudly. "And it works. If you follow the rules. So now run down and up the stairs."

He didn't budge from the bed. "There isn't any more cheesecake so what's the point?"

I poked his rounded belly and said, "That's the point."

The next time he asked for a piece of cheesecake, I left only a small bite on a plate upstairs. "What's this?" he complained. "Where's the rest of it?"

"Downstairs on the counter." I'd left a second small bite there for him to find after he climbed down the stairs. He went down and stared at the small square. Before he could protest, I reminded him about the rule. "You can have another bite upstairs."

"This is ridiculous. I'm not going to go up and down the stairs to eat a piece of cheesecake."

"See." I felt triumphant. "It works!"

We both lost 10 pounds, thanks to my trick. But although he's lighter, he's a bit crabbier. I'm coming up with another trick to take care of that.

~Lori Phillips

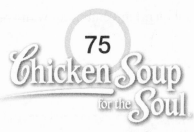

75

Lip Service

*Nothing would be more tiresome than eating and drinking
if God had not made them a pleasure as well as a necessity.*

~Voltaire

When I was a child, my mother taught me to say grace before eating a meal. That was one of her house rules. I'd whisper: "Bless us oh Lord and these thy gifts which we are about to receive from thy bounty...." Through the years I'd always done that without fail—my brain sometimes on autopilot. One day, in a moment of perfect clarity, I actually took the time to look at the "meal" I was about to consume and made an interesting discovery: not one item on the plate in front of me came from nature's bounty at all. That was my ah-ha moment.

On the spot, I started recording every morsel I could remember ingesting that week. That simple diary revealed nothing but processed, pre-packaged fare loaded with artery-clogging trans fats and artificial ingredients I couldn't even pronounce. I had been consuming a cornucopia of candy bars, corn dogs, colas and deep-fried pastries. I couldn't recall the last time I had actually consumed anything that was truly a raw, living food occurring naturally in nature. My body had ballooned to a whopping 160 pounds, and I was often tired, out of sorts and languishing from some non-specific malaise. At that moment, I resolved to redeem some of those "gifts" that were available to me in nature's bountiful supply—to at least be true to myself and to the childhood prayer I had been parroting all those years.

To my amazement, I discovered a totally new section of the

supermarket where living food not only resided but abounded: melons at their peak of ripeness, beautifully textured squash and pumpkins all vibrantly alive and brimming from a brilliant palette of colors that screamed at me to be eaten. Hadn't I been in this store countless times? Had I been too busy ransacking the snack aisle to even notice? At home, I inventoried my fridge, evicting the frozen pizzas and other sodium-laden mystery food that had taken up residence there. I purged my pantry, slam-dunking the carbonated sugary sodas and replacing them with natural juices and herbal teas.

I started experimenting with different spices and herbs. Like the French, I learned to let food linger on my tongue for a while — to actually taste and then chew fully, rather than wolfing it down my gullet like I usually did. I learned to savor the deliciousness — in short, to be in the moment with my dining experience. I learned to grill vegetables, to slather them with natural spices to enhance their flavor instead of the sour cream and butter that had been my MO. My kitchen sprang alive with fragrant fresh herbs and seasonings, citrusy and woodsy scents. I was overwhelmed that I had never appreciated this simplicity before. Another payoff: my overall digestion improved and I started sleeping more soundly at night. Before long I had whittled 25 pounds off my body and four inches from my waistline!

I began to value the awesome design of raw vegetables and fruits, to enjoy them in their entirety, skins and all, their natural sheaths loaded with flavor and nutrients. I marveled at the unique beauty inherent in their patterns — in their very DNA. By replanting the seeds hidden inside them, I was able to reproduce for another day the unadulterated goodness I had just consumed. From my humble garden, I began to reap the benefits of a more healthful diet, and the pounds continued to drop off. Finally, I learned to accept the gifts from nature that had always been accessible to me — I just had never slowed down long enough to observe and relish. My humble garden provided not only a harvest of nourishment, but a haven of serenity and quiet reflection.

Along with exercise and sleeping more soundly, I began to morph into a more alert, focused individual, my once nutrition-deprived brain now fully engaged and relieved of its often debilitating brain fog. Too often breakfast had either been totally non-existent or a quick powdered donut. Lunchtime meant scurrying to the nearest fast food drive-thru to snag something—anything—on the fly so I could race back to my desk job; dinner was often a delivered pizza devoured at home in front of my laptop. Now, in my newly refocused world, I started to put more deliberate effort into planning my meals. I stopped limiting myself to pre-packaged snack attack foods that were filling me out and not up.

Before eating, I still offer that same childhood blessing, but the words resonate with new meaning. Now I have an acute awareness that food represents health for my body—not a quick fix to ease some momentary ennui. Now every food I eat is "comfort" food because I'm more in sync with the very source that provided it, and I bestow honor in the way I receive that gift. I have repositioned fruits and vegetables at the core of my eating, while still enjoying meat, but in much smaller portions. I still indulge in that occasional decadent chocolate treat, but, surprisingly, it takes less of it to satisfy me. More importantly, I am in the moment with my universe and the gifts that have already been provided for me in abundance, naturally occurring and right there for the taking. A childhood blessing mouthed in haste—no longer lip service, has evolved into a daily prayer of thanksgiving.

~Elaine K. Green

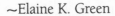

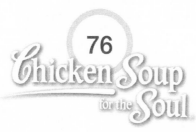

76

How Much Does a Secret Weigh?

Life itself is the proper binge.
~Julia Child

Rising off my knees and flushing the toilet, I rinsed my mouth over and over again. Bitter acid stung my throat and tears burned my cheeks. As if it weren't enough to be consumed by self-loathing, I wondered if the thin walls of my apartment would betray me. Did my roommates hear the retching, the toilet, and the water? Having started in college, I was already well-practiced at making myself throw up; I now had eight years under my belt—enough practice that I would sometimes spontaneously regurgitate if I'd eaten too much, but in this tiny apartment it was getting harder and harder to conceal my disgusting secret.

"Aaah!" I screamed into my pillow to muffle the sound. "This is insane; I am twenty-six years old and at the mercy of a stupid box of cookies." I bolted from the bed and raced into the kitchen. Seizing the three-pound half-eaten box of chocolate wafers, as if it were some living demonic force, I crushed and twisted it, my knuckles turning red, then white, with a fury that belied the happy-go-lucky person everyone else saw. After it was all over, I took the wreckage to the garbage chute and listened as it plunged 15 floors and landed with a thud. This is my life's metaphor, I thought. I've hit bottom.

I've always believed there are no coincidences, so when I saw the ad for the "Thin Within" workshop starting in two days I knew it was speaking to me.

When I arrived, I faced a room full of people obviously much heavier than I. People who wore their weight on the outside; mine was hiding within.

"What are you doing here?" the large woman sitting next to me said. "I'd love to be your size. What are you—about a 4?"

The moderator asked people to stand and state their goals for the workshop.

"Seventy pounds," called a man with double crutches. "The weight's killing my knees." "Fifteen pounds," said another woman. "I want to lose my baby weight—my baby's graduating from college in June."

I rose from my seat and stood quietly. Gripping the chair in front of me, I choked on the words, but let the tears run.

"I want to stop throwing up."

I had never said those words—to myself or to anyone else. Now before a crowd of strangers I let go of the ugly festering secret that weighed me down more than anything. The room broke into applause and the large woman sitting next to me squeezed my hand.

Every Monday for six consecutive weeks I returned to the group eager to take the next step. There were no diets, no calorie counting, and no lectures on nutrition. I knew all that stuff anyway; ironically I was a nutrition major in college. Instead we promised for the first week simply to sit down when we ate and not do anything else—no TV, no reading, no standing at the counter, just sit and eat.

The next week we rated our hunger on a scale from 1-10 with 10 being very full. We assessed our hunger before we actually ate anything and committed to eating to a 5 or 6 and then stopping. We could still eat anything we wanted, we just had to sit down and eat until we were sated not stuffed. I was resetting my appestat (that internal regulator of appetite control) that I had badly damaged with bingeing and purging. We kept diaries of what we ate and when and then we wrote letters to ourselves and others about forgiveness, love and acceptance.

I found out it wasn't weight that I was losing, but hate. How much does a secret weigh? I had grown a protective layer of fat that insulated me from dealing with my feelings; each week as I shed that protective layer I gained something else — self-acceptance.

Twenty-four years have passed since I made the promise to stop throwing up. Now at 50, I am more healthy and fit than I was in my 20s; but still I binge and purge. It's no longer the food though, but the negative self-talk and destructive criticisms that ran constantly in my head like Muzak. As for binges, those I allow — frequent and copious binges on kindness, compassion and compliments.

~Tsgoyna Tanzman

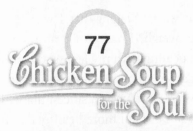

77

Eating My Idols

Prayer may not change things for you,
but it for sure changes you for things.
~Samuel M. Shoemaker

As I flipped through the pictures of my husband's retirement ceremony, I cried. The woman in the photos didn't even look like me. Over John's 20 years in the Navy, I had gained and lost over 300 pounds. Sometimes it takes the objective view of a camera lens to make us realize how we truly appear to others. I masked this last gain of 60 pounds under oversized sweaters and baggy pants until the person smiling at me from the photographs was a stranger. As I contemplated which diet to try this time, God seemed to tell me it wasn't only a diet I needed, but a change of heart as well.

The first step was to enroll in a diet center that concentrated not only on weight loss, but in teaching me how to cook and eat correctly. When I came home with my new food list, I broke into tears. I paid too much money to eat so little. I shook the offending paper in front of my bewildered husband.

"There's no way I can do this! I don't even like vegetables."

John gave me a hug and reminded me he'd support whatever I decided, but we both knew I had to at least make a valiant attempt to stick to it. I went to bed depressed and set for failure.

The next morning I woke up and found a note card on top of my Bible. On it was a verse I had written the day before. "Be strong and courageous, and do the work. Do not be afraid or discouraged by the size of the task, for the Lord, my God, is with you. He will not fail you or forsake you. He will see to it that all the work related to the Temple of the Lord is finished correctly." (1 Chr. 28:20 NLT.) I knew immediately that I was the temple of the Lord. Losing weight was more than a diet, it was a test. A test the Teacher would help me pass.

Through Bible study and prayer I realized how I had used food as an idol in my life. I'd heard the idea before, how anything we turn to instead of Christ is an idol, but now God gave me a clear vision of exactly how I glorified food. I might as well have carved out tiny statues and placed them in a shrine where I could worship them each day. A bag of potato chips represented my god of anger. A chocolate chip cookie symbolized my god of joy. Miniature idols of macaroni and cheese and pizza sat proudly on the altar of my heart and rejoiced each time I turned to them instead of the Lord. Every celebration came with cake. Doughnuts eased any disappointments. Only after I'd satisfied my food idols did I turn to the Lord in prayer. But our God is a jealous God, and he was no longer willing to take second place.

The Lord commanded, "You shall have no other gods before me." Food had crept into my heart and pushed Him out. Not completely, but enough so I turned to its seductive satisfaction first, instead of trusting completely in God and his plan for me. Through prayer I learned to give even the smallest aspects of my life to God and deny food the opportunity to lead me astray. It hasn't been easy. When the stress of work or raising teenagers overwhelms me I'm still tempted to turn to a bowl of ice cream for comfort. But even though I walk through the Valley of the Häagen-Dazs I know my God is with me. He longs to pick me up and set me back on His path again.

The journey to lose weight has been an amazing one. I feel like the Israelites being led out of Egypt, free after years of serving a foreign master. Physically, I lost over 40 pounds, started exercising regularly and even learned to like vegetables; but the spiritual results are far more rewarding. I feel God's pleasure at my obedience to his will, and that is more satisfying than any mouthful of food has ever been.

~Kim Stokely

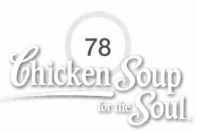

78

Taken by Surprise

Don't dig your grave with your own knife and fork.
~English Proverb

Have you ever been socked in the stomach with a doubled-up fist? You reel with shock, then catch your breath and make an effort to deal with whatever caused the wallop. It's the same when a completely unexpected health issue comes up.

On returning from vacation, I found a letter with results from a blood test. Everything was good with one exception. My doctor had ordered a fasting glucose test to be included after I'd discussed my concern over weight I'd gained. On checking my records, he expressed surprise that I'd gained 20 pounds in a two-year period. My eating habits had not changed, but I had not been as physically active, and I wondered if that could be the problem.

"Let's check your glucose and thyroid," he said, adding two more items to the list of routine things checked in a blood test.

I left the lab that day with the only reminder being the Band-Aid on my arm where the technician had drawn a sample. Then I promptly forgot about it.

Now, I looked at the number by the fasting glucose test. Just under 115 and next to it, the doctor had written "I want this number below 100!!!! You can do this by losing weight, increasing exercise, and watching foods like potatoes, bread, and pasta. We'll repeat the test in six months."

Those four exclamation marks gave me that hard sock in the

stomach. Had he ended his sentence with a period, I might not have taken the news quite as seriously. Much later, I felt most grateful that he had written his note in a way that made me sit up and pay attention.

I read health-related articles frequently, so I knew that the number indicated pre-diabetes. No one in my immediate family had been diabetic. What else might have brought it on? What part of my lifestyle had caused it? Why me?

I realized I needed to do some research and learn more about this condition, and I began that day. I learned about the risk factors, about the myths of pre-diabetes and diabetes, about the kind of diet and activity that might help me keep from progressing to Type 2 diabetes.

My two biggest risk factors were most likely having hypertension and being physically inactive for two years because of a foot problem. And, I had to admit that my favorite foods are all high in carbohydrates. At this point, I knew what I had and perhaps what brought it on.

What to do about it became the starred item on my mental list. I read about diabetic diets, bought a diabetic cookbook and studied the recipes, worrying at how deprived I might feel if I had to give up many foods I liked. I told my husband that I wasn't going to start eating a new way quite yet. First, I had to come to terms with the idea of this new condition, and I spent a full week doing just that. This condition had sneaked up and taken me by surprise. There were moments when anger washed over me, while at other times I told myself how fortunate I was that it was only pre-diabetes. I had time to do something about it. How could I feel anything other than glad that I'd had this warning sign?

I knew that making a big lifestyle change doesn't happen overnight. I began taking a daily walk, 20 minutes to begin with. It was not an enjoyable 20 minutes as I huffed and puffed with every slight incline. "Out of shape" were the three words that rolled through my mind as I walked the lovely trail that runs near our home. Day by day, I watched as spring wildflowers bloomed, and buds on trees opened into full leaves. I increased the amount of time each week, and after a full month, I was up to 40 minutes and breathed more easily. Best of all, I enjoyed the exercise, and the words that ran through my mind had changed to "This can help."

My husband had had a serious heart attack several years earlier, and I'd done a lot of reading about cardiac diets at that time. I also took advantage of a wonderful service offered at our local hospital. The Diet and Nutrition Specialist conducted classes for recent cardiac patients and their spouses. In one day with her, I learned a lot, but one of the most important things was that you don't just diet, you make a lifestyle change that must last forever. I learned to cook with less fat, cut our portion sizes, and switched to more wholegrain foods. We both lost weight with the diet and exercise program we followed, but little by little I'd slipped back into old habits. Plus I had to give up walking for exercise when my foot problem became too painful.

Now, the time had come to adhere to those rules I'd learned but forgotten, or ignored. My diet changes felt a little drastic at first. I reduced both sugar and carbohydrates, not completely, but by a great deal. I also cut the portion sizes of everything, trying to basically eat half of what I had been eating. Instead of an eight-ounce steak, I had four ounces. Instead of a bowl of cereal and a muffin or piece of coffeecake, I had cereal with fresh fruit in it. Instead of bread, I ate a couple of whole grain crackers. Instead of two cookies with afternoon tea, I had a piece of fruit. Every few days, I did have a cookie, but only one. And when I went out for lunch or dinner, I tried to order healthy food and ate half of what was brought to me, taking half home for another meal. Even when going to a friend's home for a bridge luncheon, I ate only a small portion of what was served and either skipped dessert or ate half the portion. It paid off, as I lost 14 pounds in six months.

The weight loss has been gratifying and the exercise is now enjoyable, but the best part came when I had a repeat fasting glucose test recently. The number had fallen to 100, not the "below 100" my doctor wanted to see but so close that I felt just plain giddy when I got the report.

I must remember to thank my doctor for using those four exclamation marks in his note to me. They made me realize this might become a serious situation if I didn't work at changing it. There are so many resources available to help me achieve my goal. I'm determined to keep working at it!!!! Don't think it can't happen to you. It's a sneaky little disease that crept up and took me by surprise.

~Nancy Julien Kopp

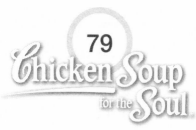

79

Weighing In

I don't run away from a challenge because I am afraid.
Instead, I run toward it because the only way to escape fear
is to trample it beneath your feet.
~Nadia Comaneci

One spring evening while I prepared dinner, my twelve-year-old daughter walked into our kitchen to find me clad only in a knit shirt, underpants and sandals. She stood in silence near the doorway observing me while I folded my capri jeans on the counter into a tiny bundle.

"What are you doing?" she asked.

"Weighing my pants," I answered while gingerly placing the strategically creased fabric on the small stainless steel platform of my food scale.

She shook her head and left the room without asking why.

The unplanned event that transpired in my kitchen had to do with my scheduled weigh-in the next morning at Weight Watchers. Every week, the day before my meeting, I'd agonize over any possible obstacle that might interfere with a positive reading the next morning. Positive would include any number that was even an ounce lower than the prior week's number.

Forget about the restaurant meal and ice cream cone that I'd had on Saturday night or the high-sodium Chinese food I'd eaten last night. The real diet buster for me that week could lie in the transition from my usual weigh-in attire. The onset of warm weather caused me to dispense with my lightweight khakis and put on a pair of denim capris, the same pants I planned on wearing the next morning to my appointment. What a waste to watch my caloric intake all week and then have a lousy pair of pants sabotage my efforts!

So, while I stood at the counter and chopped broccoli, all the while considering tomorrow's fateful event, I eyed the small food scale. Without missing a beat, I dropped my knife, pushed aside the broccoli and removed my pants. Even my daughter's judgmental stare couldn't stop me.

I made a note of the number, but it didn't end with the capris.

A comparison to the previously worn weigh-in attire was necessary, so I slipped on my pants and took the food scale up to my bedroom.

Once upstairs, the diet con artist in me took over. I decided to check out several items in the hopes of locating outfits that were lighter than what I wore the prior weeks. With this strategy, weight loss could occur without a single change in my caloric intake. I folded shirts and bras into tiny packages that could fit on the scale's platform. I even checked my underpants and jewelry. The only thing I didn't weigh was myself!

But in the middle of comparing the meager one-ounce difference between two pairs of earrings, I stopped. What was I doing?

I'd been on diets since the age of fifteen, and was now fifty. There was one thing that remained consistent in that period of time; I was scared stiff of knowing my weight!

In fact, my fear of the scale was part of the reason I'd lose 15 or 20 pounds and then put it right back on six months later. After almost every weight loss I'd ever achieved, if the button on my pants felt a little snug, rather than boldly stepping up to the plate and assessing the damage, I'd ignore it.

My ingenious plan always involved losing the weight first and then weighing myself. Similar to how young children cover their eyes and believe you can't see them, I concluded that if I didn't know the number on the scale, then it didn't exist. But the pants would stay tight, and get tighter until the day when I could no longer button them. Then I'd finally step on the scale. It was never good news.

The real root of my problem was plain and simple: fear. So, against all sound diet advice I'd ever read, heard on TV or was told by friends, I decided there was only one way to get over this fear.

I began to weigh myself every single day as soon as I got up.

Even on a day after I'd gone to a party and stuffed myself.

Even on a day when I had to loosen the button on my pants while I sat at my computer the night before.

And even on the day after I'd eaten the saltiest food possible and knew I was retaining more water than a swimming pool.

Every morning I'd shut off my alarm, roll out of bed and land directly on the scale. When the number was up a pound or two, my goal would be to have it slowly go down before it got any higher.

That was a year ago. I've been through Halloween, Thanksgiving and Christmas. While there have been days when I've gained a few of my lost pounds back, the daily reminder makes me get myself in check much faster than my previous avoidance technique. And, usually, the small weight gains disappear in a few days. Much easier than trying to lose the full 15 or 20 pounds all over again.

My fear has subsided, too. I easily step on the scale without the dread that had previously consumed me. I may not always be happy with the outcome. Yet, I've learned to accept it's just a number and instead give myself credit for the courage it took to get on the scale in the first place.

As far as my daughter goes, I figure the incident about her pantless neurotic mother will be a story for her future therapist.

And, in case you're wondering, the denim capris weighed a pound and a half, but the khakis were only a pound and quarter.

~Sharon A. Struth

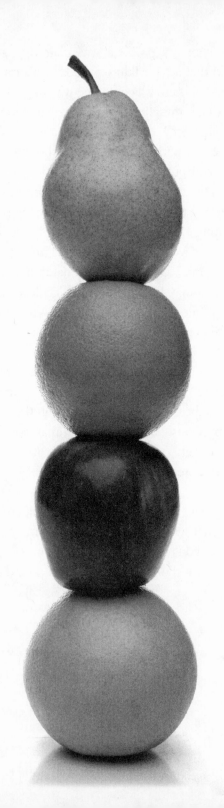

Chapter 9

Shaping the New You

Foods that Made a Difference

Food is not my enemy and I will not fear it.
I will make food my body's friend,
not its foe.

~*Richard Simmons*, The Book of Hope

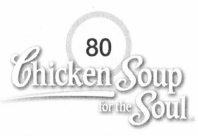

80

Soul Food

If junk food is the devil, then a sweet orange is as scripture.
~Audrey Foris

t was more than 20 years ago. I was on the couch, making a shopping list, holding my baby who almost always had an ear infection, and pretending I wasn't starting to come down with yet another bout of strep throat. That's when the one person I definitely did not want to see came over. In walked Debbie, the "natural" fanatic. I was in no mood to get a sermon about how everybody in my family was getting sick so often because I was doing everything wrong.

I tried to sit up and look perky, but I shouldn't have even wasted the little energy I had left. There was no fooling Debbie. She was adept at spotting all things phony.

Debbie knew I was getting sick again, and I think she must have also known that I was getting sick of her standard sermons. She had a different tactic this time. It was just one innocent question.

"When was the last time you ate an apple?" she asked.

I was relieved. "Apples? We've got plenty! Just check my fridge. My kids eat them all the time."

"That's not what I asked," she said, not even smiling. "I asked when was the last time you ate an apple. I'm not asking for a lot. Just one simple, unadulterated apple. Think about it. Do you enjoy getting sick so often? Why not try something you could enjoy a lot more?" And she was out the door.

I sat there fuming. But years later I found out she was a true friend.

I can still remember the taste of that first apple I bit into... years after our conversation. It wasn't as boring as I thought it would be. It tasted weird at first. Weird to be eating something so basic. Then juicy. Then delicious.

"An apple a day keeps the doctor away" is something I had heard many times, but I never understood its many ramifications. It's not just about apples. It goes for bananas as well. And peaches and oranges. Strawberries, cantaloupe—even kiwis! It goes for the infinite number of gifts God has personally packaged for us. Individually packaging each one, no less! They are all designed to help us stay well.

And what do we do with His gifts? Pass right by them, and head straight for the peach ice cream for us, and the strawberry "fruit" bars for our children.

We all too often prefer the stuff that's been taken out of its original packaging, "processed" until it's just about unrecognizable, thrown in with a few additives here, some preservatives there, artificial coloring all over the place, and voilà—we then consider it edible!

By putting our physical selves in tune with our spiritual selves—the way they were meant to be, we can spend a lot less time in the kitchen trying to "fix up" what God has already made wonderful. God's candy comes bite-sized (grapes, berries), individually packaged (nectarines, bananas, plums) and even family-sized (watermelons)—pre-prepared for our optimum health and pleasure. We need to re-learn what we once knew—how to appreciate life's simple and genuine joys.

Sure, Man cannot live on fruit alone—but there isn't a better way to start the day than by having a breakfast of fruit. Then, for the rest of the day, if we make some small effort to eat food that's still packed with Divine sparks of God's loving kindness toward us—so much the better.

We don't have to banish all the so-called "goodies" from our shelves. But every effort made in this direction can help draw us closer to God, leaving less of the distracting (and debilitating) fluff between us and Him. It can take a while to re-develop appreciation, but as the satisfaction we get from sustenance that is closer to its natural state increases, the "draw" of the "less-well-connected" food-stuffs painlessly diminishes.

You walked out my door more than 20 years ago, Debbie. And soon after that, we moved away. Then so did you. We've lost touch with each other, and I never got to tell you that I really wasn't a hope-less case, doomed to donuts and ear infections, processed "cheese food" and strep throat for the rest of my life. I am still here on the couch, writing another one of my shopping lists, but, oh boy, is it a different kind of shopping list.

Oh, you planted a seed in me alright, Debbie. Knowing you, it must have been an apple seed.

~Bracha Goetz

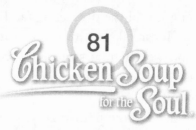

81

No Meat for Me, Thanks

Nothing will benefit human health and increase chances for survival of life on Earth as much as the evolution to a vegetarian diet.

~Albert Einstein

One hundred fifty, 160, 170... I jumped off my white bathroom scale before its flaming red pointer had the chance to deliver its final verdict. I had already seen enough.

The scale and I had first become enemies when at the age of six it was determined that what had once been affectionately called my "baby fat" was really just plain old fat. My trim mother consulted our pediatrician about my inability to lose the stubborn weight. After prodding my soft belly and considering my eating habits, the doctor determined that I needed to eat a diet laden with meat. My appetite would be satisfied by meat and I would be less apt to fill up on starchy foods like rice, pasta, and potatoes, the foods I loved. Those were the foods, he explained, that contained useless calories and made a little girl like me fat.

Long before the high protein-low carbohydrate diet was a glimmer in Dr. Atkins' unclogged arteries, my pediatrician must have seemed like a real forward thinker, and following his instructions, my family cowered before the carbohydrate, the devil's food. All vestiges of starch were removed from our pantry with the exception of bread. My father couldn't live without it and where else, he argued, would we place all our fat-fighting luncheon meats?

Meat and I were never a love match. Yet prompted by my pediatrician's recommendations, there were burgers for breakfast, pork chops for lunch, and pot roasts for dinner. My belly became bloated. My arms and legs felt sluggish. I was miserable. I was constipated. And on top of that, I was still gaining weight.

I'm not exactly sure what the food pyramid looked like back then, but even as a child I innately knew that this wasn't a good lifestyle for me. First of all, my little body wasn't faring too well trying to digest all that animal protein. Second, and perhaps more importantly, the menu was just not pleasing to the palate. There was a whole range of foods out there and I wanted them. One evening, with a brown hunk of beef laid before me, I threw myself down on the ground and simply refused to eat my dinner. Quietly, my mother removed my plate and replaced it with a bowl of blissfully buttered mashed potatoes. Diet over.

I continued to struggle with my weight throughout my childhood and in my teen years I managed to diet and exercise myself from obese to just overweight. Too often, I heard the siren song of sweet snacks, starches, and fried foods. My weight inevitably would rise as a result of these falls from grace and the diet would be over once again. As difficult as such a regimen was to maintain, I knew that the only way to a healthy weight was through a balance of fruits, vegetables, and meats.

"Not necessarily," said my friend Suzanne. Suzanne was a single mother of four teenage boys who worked with me full time and went to college at night. She was tall and slender with shiny brown hair and clear skin, a picture of health and energy. And she was a vegetarian.

"I don't eat anything with a face," she joked as she ran some cabling from my PC to my new printer. "That's how I stay in shape."

"But you must have been slim your whole life," I countered as I twisted to remove my ample hips from my office chair. "I've had a weight problem my whole life. Giving up meat wouldn't ever get me in the type of shape you're in."

Suzanne turned toward me, serious. "You didn't know me back then," she said. "I was a mess. I would balloon up, then starve myself.

After the birth of my youngest, nothing worked. I was in such bad shape that all I did was lie on the sofa and listen to radio talk shows." Suzanne went on to explain that she started to become interested in one of the health and fitness shows that promoted a vegetarian life style. That was one eating program she hadn't yet tried. Me neither. But, I was willing to give it a shot.

So, armed with a jiggly block of beige tofu and a few recipes from Suzanne, I became a vegetarian and amazing things started happening. I started to lose weight and I had more energy. Exercise was no longer a chore, but a pleasure. Before long I had shiny hair and a glowing complexion, like my mentor. Let me be perfectly clear here; this was not the result of simply eliminating meat from my diet. Suzanne had recommended several books about the benefits of a diet filled with fresh fruits and vegetables, whole grains, and plant-based proteins like soy and legumes. I bought the books, studied them carefully, weighed the pros and cons, then with the blessing of my doctor, followed a program that appeared to be medically sound. I started to become really involved in what I ate and delighted in making new discoveries about food. For example, shredded zucchini can make a very tasty and filling substitute for spaghetti. I found that I actually preferred sweet potatoes to French fries and veggie burgers to cheeseburgers. Cooking became an adventure and I sometimes even baked my own grain breads. I know that sounds time-consuming, however I found my new hobby relaxing.

Even though I sometimes enjoyed a cookie or half a doughnut with my afternoon tea, I eventually reached my goal weight. That's when I had the pleasure of replacing my entire wardrobe. My feet no longer ached and my hips no longer stuck to the side of theater seats. Finally, I was free! Yet, the crowning moment came when I made my annual visit to the doctor. I watched proudly as the scale's pointer came to rest on an acceptable number. In her office later, my doctor reviewed my records: blood pressure, good; cholesterol, good. She peered at me over her reading glasses. Weight, good. My body mass index, she told me, was smack dab in the middle of the medically recommended range.

"That's what happens," said Suzanne, "because being a vegetarian is a lifestyle, not a diet. Diets fail because they're only a temporary way of eating, but this is a total commitment to healthier living."

Even though I'm a success story, I understand that becoming a vegetarian is not for everyone. I suspect that any eating program that advocates a wide variety of healthy foods eaten in moderate portions can be equally as successful. As for me, however, when the platter of meat is passed around the dinner table, I just recall the miserable six-year-old girl, the plump teenager, or the frustrated adult I once was and say, "No meat for me, thanks. I'll pass."

~Monica A. Andermann

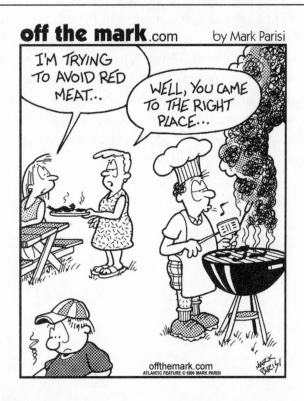

Reprinted by permission of Off the Mark
and Mark Parisi ©1996

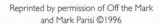

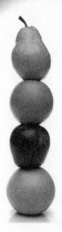

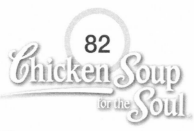

82

The Power of Words

To keep the body in good health is a duty...
otherwise we shall not be able to keep our mind strong and clear.
~Buddha

Have you ever read a quote or phrase that made such a profound impression on you that it changed your life? That's what happened to me when I encountered two powerful truths about nutrition and exercise. The impression these words made on me was so strong that I changed my eating habits and my commitment to exercise.

I had always read articles on nutrition and exercise and was educated on how important both are to good health. My problem wasn't that I lacked information, but that I hadn't acted upon the information I had. I wasn't sure how to go from "knowing" to "doing"—that was until I read some powerful words.

While thumbing through *Natural Health* magazine, I came upon three simple words—"Food is medicine." This simple phrase resonated so powerfully within me, that it changed how I looked at food. I thought about every morsel I put in my mouth and realized that each bite was medicine that would affect my body for good or for bad. Eating was like taking a dose of medicine. If I wanted good health, then I needed to take the right medicine.

I believed that if I changed only one important aspect of my diet it would support my new philosophy. I stopped eating foods with preservatives. I saw preservatives as bad medicine—chemicals that would ultimately harm my body just like a wrong prescription from the pharmacy. If I couldn't pronounce an ingredient on a package or didn't have a clue what it was, I didn't dare put it in my mouth. All natural foods were good medicine. This resulted in a diet of fresh meats, fruits and vegetables. When I wasn't buying produce, I looked for packaged items that boasted of having no preservatives.

Within a month, I saw a dramatic change in my body. My complexion was clear and smooth. I had more energy, and I felt good. I even slept better. As an added bonus, I dropped five pounds. I was taking good medicine for my body at every meal, and I was experiencing the benefits of good health.

A quote, by Edward Stanley, changed my attitude about exercise because it appealed to my conviction about the importance of planning for retirement. I had always been taught to save money for my "golden years," but Stanley's words made me realize how important it was to bank good health. "Those who think they have not time for bodily exercise will sooner or later have to find time for illness." Wow! That hit me right in the IRA—Internal Response Adjuster. If I didn't make time for exercise now, then I'd have to make time for illness later.

I knew that I had to begin preparing my health for the future. My past attempts at staying committed to exercise had failed, so I needed to come up with a plan to stay consistent. I planned to exercise first thing in the morning before the distractions of the day began. I figured that I'd have to get up at 5:30 a.m. in order to exercise for 45 minutes, shower and get my son to school on time. My exercise program consisted of 30 minutes of walking on my treadmill and five minutes of stretching. After stretching, I spent the last 10 minutes doing either yoga, Pilates or free weights. I alternated between those three during the week for variety in my routine. On mornings when the alarm rang and I didn't want to get out of bed to exercise, I kept repeating to myself, "I'm investing in my future, I'm investing my future." Unlike the recent stock market, I knew my exercise program would give me a substantial return on my investment.

The habit of exercising Monday through Friday has been one of the best things I've ever done for myself. Exercising early in the morning to avoid interruptions, and my new philosophy of investing in my future health, have kept me committed and consistent. I use the weekends as a reward to sleep late and rest my body. I've never felt or looked better.

Two simple phrases, profound truths, changed the way I thought about nutrition and exercise. The power of those words inspired me to eat better and make exercise a habit. As a result, I'm enjoying healthy days now and looking forward to healthy days to come.

~Debbie Cannizzaro

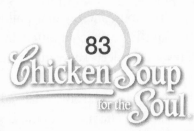

83

Listening to My Body

Sometimes your body is smarter than you are.

~Author Unknown

Recently while hiking in the Austrian Alps, I misread the signs and ended up taking a trail that grew more and more challenging, eventually becoming so steep that my body couldn't go any farther. It simply gave up. Exhausted and lost, with crumbling scree beneath me and slippery rocks above, my body forced me to accept the fact that I was on the wrong path.

Hanging there, clutching a few slick blades of grass and loose rocks that no wise man would have built a house on, I had a few minutes to think about another time when my body had given up on me.

It all started 15 years ago when I moved from my hometown in Tennessee to the home of bread and beer: Munich, Germany. My life was about to take a turn, and not for the better. At first I was overwhelmed by the adventure of it all: a new country, a new job, a new relationship, new pain.

Yes, pain. The second I got off the plane in Munich, I was introduced to delicious, dark bread and German beer—which the Bavarians call "liquid bread"—and I enthusiastically took up the tradition of eating a pretzel with cold butter each morning. I also got my fork into a few *Semmelknödel*, an unimpressive, soggy ball of boiled bread (but it sure was good for sopping up tasty gravy). The food was really great, but slowly my body began to sense that something was really wrong.

It took me, at least the thinking part of me, five more years to understand what was happening. In my defense, I didn't notice overnight that I was climbing up the wrong path. My diet in Nashville had rarely included bread or pretzels or anything spelled with an umlaut. I didn't like beer, and I'd even had the good sense to stop eating pasta 20 years ago when I realized it caused bloating. In the years before I moved to Munich, I'd had bread on occasion, so I'd been experiencing minor intestinal worries off and on for quite some time. Also in my defense, I'm afraid of doctors—which, admittedly, is more of a cop-out than a defense.

In 2001, my body was in such bad shape that it needed a doctor. I had shingles—at the age of thirty-seven. My immune system was exhausted. My body simply couldn't continue on the same path. It was time to face facts, but first I had to find them. I typed my symptoms—fatigue, joint pain, nausea, regular intestinal irregularity, bloating, and irritability, among a few others—into as many Internet search engines as I could find. This was very helpful. As it turned out, it seemed I had my pick of every trendy ailment in the book, from fibromyalgia to mad cow disease.

One search result, however, kept rearing its glutenous head: an intolerance to gluten, the protein found in wheat, barley, rye and possibly oats. Remembering my bout with pasta 20 years ago, I said to my body, "Ah-ha!" and went on a gluten-free diet. (If you suspect gluten or celiac disease might be your problem but you love Italian food, you'll want to be 100 percent sure before you change your life. Go to your doctor and ask to be tested.)

The diet was no walk in the park at first. I had to start by figuring out what all those letters and numbers on labels stand for. Who knows what lurks behind those E541-like abbreviations anyway? I do… now. A man obsessed, I refused to eat anything with even a trace of gluten in it.

Dinner invitations posed a minor problem—"minor" only because I don't have many friends who'd invite me to dinner. The long-suffering saints who did invite me, however, were eager to support me in my experiment. Yet even after my fascinating, two-hour lecture on the benefits of a gluten-free diet—in which I explained repeatedly that gluten is found only in wheat, barley, rye and maybe oats—one friend still asked, "Can you eat rice?"

"Well, yes," I said with a straight face, "if it's the kind of rice that doesn't have wheat, barley, rye or maybe oats in it."

"Good point! Let me check the label," she said and trotted off to the kitchen.

During dinner, the same person kept passing me the breadbasket and squinting maliciously. I know she was trying to poison me. I couldn't blame her: I had asked her to check the label on the potatoes after she checked the rice. Everyone else at the table thought it was funny. The point is, most people don't know what to do with the word "gluten." It sounds as if it should be in sticky rice and Elmer's glue, which I haven't eaten since second grade.

Bread, liquid and solid, was not easy to give up in a city with a bakery on every corner and a brewery in between. Still, I persisted in turning my diet around. Since moving to Munich, I hadn't had my mother's cornbread, so I called home for the recipe I was raised on. I discovered an organic bakery in Munich that bakes gluten-free breads from amaranth, quinoa and rice. The only friend I mourned was my daily pretzel with cold butter. Thinking now about a *Butterbrez'n* makes my mouth—and eyes—water.

After a grueling three months of careful label reading and boring my friends to death with the latest in gluten-free trivia, my body and the thinking part of me had another "Ah-ha!" moment. We were symptom-free. The intestinal worries had stopped almost immediately. I no longer felt as if someone had blown up my belly with a bicycle pump. My morning nausea had vanished with the *Butterbrez'n*. I dropped 10 pounds once I dropped the beer. My joints had stopped hurting. Granted, I was still irritable, but that's just me.

Today, I'm so grateful to finally know what was causing my health problems. I've been on a gluten-free path for years now. Of course, I might have avoided the pain of shingles if I had read the signs correctly that my body already understood 15 years ago. But without the knowledge that something as wholesome as wheat and barley could make me sick, I had to learn the hard way—just like I had to do in the Austrian Alps, holding on for dear life near the top of what turned out to be a waterfall.

I hung there for an embarrassingly long time before I mustered the courage to crawl, slide and tumble back down. An elderly Austrian man at the bottom—I'm sure he was a doctor—told me later that even if I had made it to the top, I'd have found only a sheer cliff with no way to get back down safely.

Once again, I was fortunate that my body had the good sense to give up when I could still get back to the right path.

~Christopher Allen

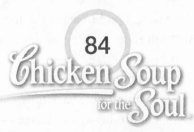

84

Blessed Beans

Mrs. Goldberg and Mrs. Weiss are lunching
at a well-known Miami Beach hotel.
"The food here is terrible," says Mrs. Goldberg.
"And such small portions!"
adds Mrs. Weiss.
~The Big Little Book of Jewish Wit & Wisdom
edited by Sally Ann Berk

"God Bless Heinz Vegetarian Beans!" I found myself saying this prayerful reflection to myself as I was about to address my congregation on the eve of Yom Kippur. Sixty-five pounds down within the year, and without a doubt my most successful daily meal was a can of Heinz Vegetarian Beans. Sometimes, I daydream that H.J. Heinz will hire me as their official rabbinic spokesman and I will become the new "Subway Jared" for this alternative magical prescription to successful weight loss. This daydream takes on many forms. My favorite is appearing on *The Oprah Winfrey Show* and commiserating with her on how hard it is to be a public figure and address one's eating problems, yo-yo weight loss and gain, etc. Oprah would embrace my new insight into the power of the "bean" and I'd solve all my financial stresses moving forward.

My daydreaming usually abruptly ends at this point. I discovered Heinz Vegetarian Beans in college because it was what I could afford to eat on a regular basis and it provided me a healthy meal. I remember being embarrassed when my wife-to-be, Roseanne, first came to the studio apartment I shared with two other roommates. She looked in my kitchen cabinet and saw stacks of cans of Heinz Vegetarian Beans. I recall how, back then, I shamefully admitted that it was what I routinely ate. But, it was also in college that I was my leanest and healthiest self. Once I started working and had easier access to funds, I don't think I ever had a can of my old favorite. And, now, with the nutritional program I had pursued, I had formally learned the power of low fat, high protein, and the wonders of hunger-fulfilling fiber. The beans that once had been my affordable fallback had now become my nostalgic source of properly proportioned and well-balanced eating.

So, I stood on the pulpit, took a big breath, and decided to confess to them my greatest challenge. They had all noticed, and many had commented on, the miraculously lost 65 pounds. I was trusting in them to share my secret. It was no miracle; it is the hardest, most difficult struggle I have ever pursued. I feel ensnared within a constant trap of mental and physical delusion, struggling daily with my overeating as addiction. I, the rabbi who assists them daily with successfully confronting challenges of faith, identity, spirituality, and connection, was only recently coming to terms with the fact that I have a terribly real personal struggle with addictive behavior. And, in fact, my professional life often acted as a catalyst to pursuing my mindless escapes with food.

I confessed that while I have no sweet tooth, portion size is my runaway train. Family legend holds that my first phrase was "French fries," although as reported to me by my parents, what I really said often as a toddler was "free fries." I recalled this fact with bittersweet humor because my escapism with food was really so much more problematic when I had the ability to freely access it.

Even my religious tradition seemingly blessed the problematic choices I was making. There is an old Jewish joke that declares: "we were persecuted; we overcame; now we eat!" The anecdotal experiences of my lifetime are that much of Jewish life often appears to revolve around the enjoyment of food. The custom of a traditional weekly Sabbath observance, in most Jewish homes, is to treat family and loved ones to mini-banquets.

Rarely is there ever an official "Jewish event" where there isn't a generous offering of delicacies to enjoy. The one major exception is Yom Kippur, our "Day of Atonement," where we observe a 24-hour fast. But, prior to this sacred fast many families and friends gather for their pre-Yom Kippur buffet. And, the break-fast after Yom Kippur is probably the single greatest sales event for bagels, cream cheese and lox of which I am aware.

I was contemplating all of this as I chose to share with my congregational family: "I am a binge eater." I also told them, "Food control is my most difficult personal daily challenge." And I confessed, "It's a billion times easier to keep kosher than to watch what I eat; I can eat as much kosher pastrami as I want, but to refrain from that which is ritually permitted, that is my constant 'stumbling block before the blind.'"

My congregational family laughed, but also they cared. And, afterwards many have come to me admitting to their own personal struggles with food or other addictive challenges that they confront. Now we talk as family, siblings who share similar challenges. We discuss how we need to acknowledge and accept that we have a problem. And then find for ourselves the support, love and compassion that can give us the strength to confront the obstacles that stand between us and our success.

It's never easy. We have to retrain our minds and be vigilant. When a wonderful spread of foods becomes magically available you have to transform your immediate instinct to prayerfully declare, "Hallelujah," into the much more serious prayerful reflection of "please help me find the strength to stick to my food plan."

When Yom Kippur concluded last year, my greatest accomplishment for the day was passing on the bagels, cream cheese and lox, and instead choosing to enjoy my can of Heinz Vegetarian Beans. I thanked God for my healthy choice and meal. And, I decided to recast the old Jewish joke into a wiser proverb: "we are eternally challenged; we can forever overcome; now let's find the best way for each individual to appropriately celebrate."

~Rabbi Mitchell M. Hurvitz

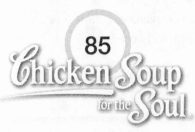

85

Dairy-Free Queen

Poets have been mysteriously silent on the subject of cheese.
~Gilbert K. Chesterton

Tears drenched my cheeks as I traveled the short distance home from the allergist. The shocking news made all the sense in the world, but my mind refused to accept it. Me, an asthmatic at the age of thirty-two? The dentist, wary about my long list of drug allergies, had insisted I see an allergist before he dared administer Novocain.

That morning in the allergist's office, after answering pages of questionnaires, the nurses had pricked and prodded me. All for a Novocain problem? Then, the breathing tests. The nurse had shaken her head and urged me to try harder the second time. I managed just under 70 percent. She explained, "Your history of bronchitis and double pneumonia this past year was a red flag for asthma. Now we've confirmed it. The good news is that you have no allergy to Novocain."

Good news? Good grief!

The nurse armed me with antihistamines and inhalers for my mold, dust mite and cat allergies. The inhaler did relieve the tightness in my chest. For the first time in a year, I felt like I could take deep breaths. Amazing that I'd gotten used to a lack of oxygen in my blood. No wonder I wanted to collapse on the couch each evening after long days with my two preschoolers.

Questions bombarded my brain. Would I always have to take medicine? Would I continue to suffer from pneumonia and bronchitis? What about our health insurance? I envisioned myself carting around an oxygen tank on my back with plastic tubes running to my nose. Would I get better?

With medication and slight changes to my environment, my health improved dramatically in a few weeks. I adjusted to the idea of taking medicine and got on with my life. Advice poured in from well-meaning family and friends, but only one comment stuck. My friend Dana shared the recommendation from her naturopath who had recently treated her young children suffering from chronic ear infections and colds. He removed all dairy foods from their diet and within weeks, they all regained their health. Without dairy products, they remained perfectly healthy.

As a child, I had some food allergies but outgrew them. I never enjoyed drinking milk, but loved ice cream, yogurt and cheese. I parked the information Dana shared with me somewhere in my memory, but didn't really give it much attention. Give up ice cream? That would be a bit drastic!

Within months, we found ourselves moving our worldly belongings across the ocean to live in The Netherlands, my husband's homeland. At the Dutch family doctor, I received ongoing treatment for my asthma, which seemed to be worsening in spite of our new mold and mildew-free living environment. About every three months, I came down with a new case of bronchitis. Instead of searching for the cause of my downward spiral, the doctor only increased the strength of my inhalers.

After a frustrating year, a nurse friend warned me, "Your lungs become damaged every time you have bronchitis and have to increase your medicine. You need to find what's causing the asthma to worsen." Once again, I pictured myself with an oxygen tank strapped to my back.

My fear turned into prayers. God, what is causing the asthma? Just tell me and I'll do whatever it takes. I don't want to end up with that tank on my back. Then, from the recesses of my mind came Dana's story about eliminating dairy.

Was that it? Did I need to eliminate all types of dairy from my diet? Impossible in Holland! This country is dairy land—the best yogurt and cheeses in the world! That would mean no more ice cream! Christmas loomed just around the corner. How could I survive the holidays without dairy? I refused to listen to those crazy thoughts.

Just days after New Year's, the doctor prescribed yet another, stronger inhaler to help clear my lungs. That potent medicine was the final straw. I made up my mind and shared my difficult decision with my husband, "Babe, I'm going to try to go off of dairy for the next eight weeks to see if my asthma improves. Will you be willing to adapt your diet in the beginning to help me out?"

"Whatever it takes, I'll help." And he meant it. He and the kids could still eat their ice cream and cheese, but all those fabulous Dutch mashed potato dishes made with creamy butter and milk would need serious adaptations.

Within two weeks, I noticed a big difference in my breathing, and by the end of eight weeks, my lungs felt open again. My energy levels increased and I suspected I had found the answer. As a small trial, on Easter, I poured yogurt dressing on my salad and treated myself to a big piece of Mont Blanc whipped cream pie. The next day I was treated to an asthma attack and flu-like symptoms when all my glands swelled. The proof was in the pudding.

From that point on, I ate dairy-free. The first six months were the most challenging. I focused on all the foods I could no longer enjoy: ice cream, chocolate, melted cheese, pizza, etc.... Life felt so unfair! Finally, I realized how many amazing dairy-free foods I could have and chose to focus on all the healthy choices I was forced to make.

I became the dairy-free queen. It required being creative and adapting my favorite recipes to be dairy-free. I scrupulously read the labels on every package and discovered the code words for hidden dairy ingredients like casein and whey. I hunted down soy and dairy-free products in the grocery and health food stores.

After three months, I stopped using my daily inhalers. For the next five years I used them only sporadically when exposed to cats or molds. In the past three years, I am happy to report that although I keep a light dosage inhaler on hand, I haven't needed it.

Right from the start of my dairy-free endeavors, I tried to reintroduce slight amounts of dairy into my diet about every six months. I knew my life would be much easier if I developed a bit of tolerance. Finally, four years ago, I found I could ingest small amounts of butter or chocolate without any adverse reactions. Chocolate! Whipped cream, ice cream and cheese are still no-no's, but I don't mind. I can eat chocolate!

Giving up dairy meant regaining my health in more ways than one. I no longer suffer from asthma, my cholesterol (genetically high) stays in a healthy range, and I can manage my weight because of all the high calorie desserts that I politely decline.

When I first said I'd do whatever it took, I'm not sure I meant it. The price of a dairy-free lifestyle seemed too high to pay. But now, the rewards far outweigh any sacrifice I've had to make.

~Johnna Stein

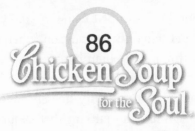

86

The Power of Oatmeal

The most indispensable ingredient of all good home cooking:
love, for those you are cooking for.
~Sophia Loren

I don't want to blame my genes for not fitting into my jeans, but one thing my Italian mother taught me was how to eat. I was a chubby kid. Every day after school, my mother had a treat waiting for me: a slice of cheesecake, almond cookies or a plate of cannolis. I sipped my first cappuccino in third grade and found the taste bitter unless accompanied by a sweet. Then, I discovered the dynamic combination of taking one sip of coffee for every bite of pastry.

Sundays were the best. That's when we had our big spaghetti dinners, and to this day my mouth waters remembering the bounty of it all. Meatballs, sausages, antipasto, and rigatoni for a pasta backup if we ran out of spaghetti. There were so many people around laughing and talking, it was easy to lose track of how much you were eating. Not that you could get away with enjoying only one plate of food. If you refused a second portion of anything, my mother's response was, "What's the matter? You don't like my cooking?"

I naturally carried this high-calorie diet into adulthood, though I rarely bothered making marinara from scratch. I could never emulate my mother's sauce. Consuming lots of breads, pasta and desserts never struck me as strange or self-indulgent; it just felt like going home.

It wasn't until I hit my mid-30s that I realized something had to change. I had little energy and, because my sluggish body didn't want to do anything, it seemed life was passing me by.

When a friend suggested I start each day with oatmeal for breakfast, I said, "You've got to be kidding!" But this friend looked great and possessed boundless enthusiasm so I took her advice.

I'm not exaggerating when I say oatmeal is one of the few dieting choices I've made to significantly change the quality of my life. It's filling without being high in calories or fat.

I used to get so hungry between breakfast and lunch, reaching for yet another cup of coffee and its charming companion, the pastry. Now, I don't even think about food until lunchtime where I pass on the pasta dishes, knowing I'll want a nap afterward.

After a year of eating oatmeal for breakfast every morning, seven days a week, I lost over 15 pounds. I have more energy to do things, like take a walk after getting home from work instead of plopping down for a snooze.

My friends and co-workers have noted the positive results of good old-fashioned oatmeal. I will admit this fundamental fiber can get boring. Try sprinkling some raisins or shaved almonds in the pot. Top it off with vanilla-flavored soy milk that's high in calcium, low in sugar and you're in for one healthy breakfast treat!

There's only one person in my life who is wary of this new diet. Every time I visit my mom, she pats me on the cheek and asks, "Honey, are you getting enough to eat?" To put her at ease, I'll pull a package of biscotti from my purse. As I sit down at a table with her and dunk one of the family favorites, I don't feel I'm cheating on my diet. Every once in a while, I just need to go home.

~Sandra Stevens

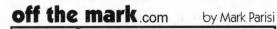

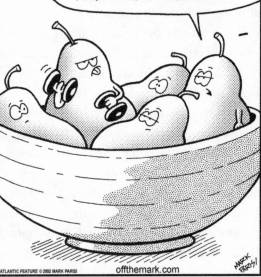

Reprinted by permission of Off the Mark
and Mark Parisi ©2002

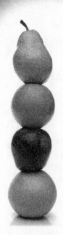

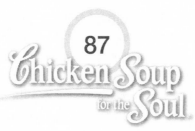

87

A Diet for Living

I may not be there yet, but I'm closer than I was yesterday.
~Author Unknown

My foot hurt as I walked to the mailbox. Confused for a moment, I stopped, stretching my right foot and testing the feel of it. Tears streamed down my face as I walked back into the house and woke my husband with a gentle shake.

"My foot hurts," I said as I woke him and in his grogginess, he simply stared, trying to figure out why this warranted waking him up early and why I was crying.

"My right foot hurts," I repeated, adding emphasis to the word "right." His eyes widened and he grinned.

"It's working?"

"It's working," I replied and sat on the edge of the bed, holding his hand and crying tears of joy.

•••

The fireplace was crackling and one of the Trans-Siberian Orchestra's Christmas albums was playing while I sat in the middle of the living room floor, merrily wrapping presents.

With a reach and a stretch, I pulled a box to me and immediately felt a twinge in my back. At thirty-two, I was young and in relatively good health, though about 30 pounds heavier than I should be, so I cringed and whined a bit about the pain, but assumed it was nothing major. Then I took some over-the-counter painkillers and went back to my Christmas preparations.

Through the holidays and into the new year, the twinge and pain continued, so in mid-January I found a chiropractor who managed to stop the pain with just a few treatments. About the same time the back pain ended, I noticed my right foot began to go numb and seemed constantly beset with pins and needles. Blaming the chiropractor, I stopped my treatment and went to see my regular physician.

Over the next several months, I had dozens of X-rays and two MRIs. I saw a back surgeon, a neurologist and more of my physician than I ever wanted to.

I raced to the doctor's office, demanding to see someone immediately, the day the nurse called and said my back X-rays showed "something." I had spina bifida occulta, a minor birth defect in my spine that had gone undiagnosed for 32 years.

The X-rays also showed I had a sixth lumbar vertebrae, when normally people have five, and the neurologist mentioned he thought I might have multiple sclerosis. I wept in terror.

By mid-summer, the doctors concluded that I had sciatica. They recommended I lose those extra 30 pounds and perhaps take up some strengthening exercises, maybe yoga or tai chi. For the occasional back spasms, they recommended muscle relaxants and pain killers.

For a while I walked and tried to lose weight, but the constant tripping and stumbling made the doctor's advice difficult to follow. Sitting on a curb with scraped hands and knees as strangers asked if I was okay proved to be too much.

Over the next few years, I packed on another 20 pounds and fought semi-regular bouts of incredible pain. I couldn't walk half a mile without stumbling.

After four years, and a bout of double vision, the original diagnosis of MS reared its ugly head again. This time the lumbar puncture proved beyond a doubt that I had multiple sclerosis.

I cried myself to sleep, convinced the diagnosis doomed me to a wheelchair or worse. I imagined drooling on myself and being unable to take care of my own needs. I also gave up on getting back into shape.

By the fall of 2009, eight years after the original problem, I had put on another 20 pounds and lived a largely sedentary life. The pins and needles had increased in my right foot, sliding up toward my knee. I couldn't put my feet together, climb stairs, or sometimes walk without watching to see where my right foot was as the synapses had slowed their communication with my brain.

Then, someone commented on an article I had written about my MS diagnosis and suggested there might be a link between MS and gluten allergies.

I might have ignored the comment, except it triggered a distant memory of a doctor mentioning when I was a teen that I might have a gluten allergy.

The reporter and investigator in me kicked in and I did some research. Dozens of personal testimonies dotted the Internet. Particularly inspiring was the story of a marathon runner who had been nearly crippled by MS until she stopped eating gluten. Six months later, she was running again.

Never a runner, I had no delusions of such a recovery, but the idea of walking through the mall without stopping to rest or tripping and falling seemed like the promise of a whole new life. I talked it over with my husband and he agreed. We would try a gluten-free diet.

• • •

On a bright and cold November morning, two weeks after purging gluten from our diet, I stepped on a stone on the way to the mailbox and my foot hurt.

As my husband held my hand and I cried, I tried to put into words what it felt like to suddenly feel my foot again. The diet gave me back a limb I had considered virtually useless.

Through the holidays we remained mostly gluten-free, and I felt the other MS symptoms begin to slip away.

For years, I had been told that a diet needs to be a life-changing event, a change in the way we eat and the way we think about eating. Cuter clothes and vague promises of better health were never what I needed to make the change work for me.

I needed measurable results and this time, I got it. I feel my foot!

I still need to work at the diet and overcome eight years of a sedentary life, but gluten-free means that I can suddenly walk down stairs without needing a handrail. The mental fear and distrust of my body lingers, so I worry about trying to run again, but each day my confidence returns a bit more as I discover I can walk without tripping or slide my feet together without looking.

This diet has changed my life. A healthier me is just the beginning.

~Lucinda Gunnin

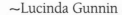

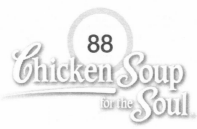

88

It's a Dog's Life

If we're not willing to settle for junk living,
we certainly shouldn't settle for junk food.
~Sally Edwards

We got our precious Corgi, Reggie, when he was just a pup. The breeder made an important request of us before signing the papers.

"If I let you have this dog," he said, "I want you to promise you won't feed him table scraps."

"What's wrong with the scraps from my table?" I replied.

"They are high in fat, calories, and processed foods, and low in nutritional value."

His response puzzled me. If my scraps were good enough for my family, they must be good enough for my pet. This made me start thinking about the quality of the food I was eating. I must admit as a teenager I easily captured the title of "Junk Food Queen." I had to change my diet at age seventeen when my doctor warned me I was headed towards Type II diabetes.

This incident with my dog made me again examine my diet. I was better than the average American—wasn't I? After all, I did not smoke, drink alcohol, or chew. Added to that, I did not eat many carbs or drink caffeine. I was looking more like a health nut every day. Upon further investigation, I realized much of what Americans consume daily is exactly what this vet challenged me to avoid for my dog. If these foods were not good enough for my dog, then they were not good enough for my family.

I was beginning to see that we have inverted the food pyramid. This contributes to our problems with heart disease, blood pressure, cancer, etc. I decided to change my diet by drinking more water, eating more fresh fruits and vegetables, eating lean meats, and further limiting fast foods. It did not take me long to feel and see the difference. My blood work was looking better with every checkup. I admit it was hard to give up the desserts and fried foods that had snuck back into my lifestyle—but what a difference it made in my health. As age creeps up on me, my health means everything. And yes, I can still occasionally eat one of those savory desserts.

I was beginning to discipline my diet when my dog taught me another lesson. At age three, my dog began to have seizures. The vet said Reggie needed medication. We increased his water intake, but never gave him the medication. We had moved to an apartment while building a new home. Our dog was cooped up all day until we got home from work, so we decided to walk him several miles daily. Several months later, I took him to the vet for his checkup.

"How are Reggie's seizures?" he asked.

"Well," I pondered, "he has not had a seizure in about… five to six months." We were so busy moving and building, I neglected to notice they had stopped.

"What has changed?" he inquired.

After thinking, I responded, "We have been exercising him each day after work, and we have been giving him more water."

"Exercise and hydration have great benefits," he explained. "Dehydration can be a cause of seizures and exercise helps to regulate chemicals in the brain. It appears this new exercise and increased water may have cured Reggie's seizures."

I began to think—if all this exercise and hydration is good enough for my dog—then surely, it is good enough for me. I researched the benefits of hydration and found this body of mine must have the right amount of water for thousands of chemical reactions to take place daily, which ensure my good health. My brain and body are comprised of 70 to 75 percent water. I was astonished to find dehydration of cells is a major cause of cancer, kidney stones, and can be a cause of seizures. Exercise also benefits the body by strengthening the heart, lungs and bones, and keeping our brains alert and healthy. We now exercise vigorously 30 to 60 minutes four to five times each week.

Reggie went to the vet for his 15-year checkup recently. The vet was amazed at how well he has done.

"He's almost ninety-nine years old in dog years," he marveled. "The average Corgi lives about 12 years. He's beating the averages."

Reggie can no longer walk several miles with us. In his older years, he can only walk about one mile without becoming exhausted. I am thankful Reggie has made it this long and retained his health. Exercise, water, and diet are clearly the reasons why. We have benefited, too. Our diets are filled with fresh fruits and vegetables, lean meats and seafood, and healthy omegas and oils. We count those glasses of water and squeeze a lemon or lime to add a little taste. We have even bought an elliptical machine so we can exercise when it is cold or raining.

My dog Reggie was actually not my first lesson in taking care of my body. My first lesson came in my childhood years when my dad worked for U.S. Senator Strom Thurmond. The Senator treated me as one of his own and constantly gave me lectures about food, diet and exercise. My third grade health book was also filled with this same information. Unfortunately, I didn't listen.

"Don't eat too much junk food," Senator Thurmond would always say. "Fruits and vegetables are God's way of keeping you healthy."

At age eighty, the Senator jogged five miles each day, worked 60 to 80 hour weeks, and kept up with his four young children. When Strom Thurmond died at age 100, the doctor signed his death certificate with these words, "Cause of Death: old age." Rarely does anyone's death certificate say that these days.

The Bible commands us to take care of our bodies. The discipline we have developed in this area has helped us to grow in mind, body, and spirit. We now look at our health in a new light. If it's good enough for my dog, it's good enough for me. Better said, I should take care of myself as least as well as I care for my dog.

~Ginny Dent Brant

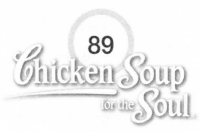

89

The Condiment Queen Clams Up

*Condiments are like old friends—
highly thought of, but often taken for granted.*
~Marilyn Kaytor

've always enjoyed a condiment or two with my meal, but I never realized they were my downfall until "the tartar sauce incident." A native New Englander, I insist that every return to the shoreline include an encounter with fried whole belly clams. Ask Connecticut friends and family my number one priority when visiting and the unanimous response is "fried clams." Fried clams are big business in Connecticut. Even in the off-peak hours, people line up at their local clam shacks for those greasy little delicacies. They are made even sweeter by a patch of tartar sauce. It's not atypical for me to use all of my tartar sauce and move on to my husband's portion.

"Why not just have a nice big bowl of tartar sauce?" my husband teased on our last visit. "Then we wouldn't have to wait in line for a table during tourist season."

I thought his comment was funny but it was also true. Was I packing on the pounds because of my vacation ration of fried foods, or had I become condiment crazy?

Upon closer examination, my mayo mania was obvious. Horseradish sauce. Blue cheese dressing. Guacamole. Clam dip. Sour cream. When I'm done, you'd be hard pressed to spot a bagel under the cream cheese or a cracker under my artichoke dip. My mantra has always been "Never skip the hollandaise." In a former life I was a sous chef, or more specifically, a saucier. A saucier is the exotic title for a sauce maker. There is no title, exotic or otherwise, for the compulsive consumer of condiments except maybe "overweight."

Armed with an awesome set of measuring spoons, I decided to meet my demons head on. Their vital statistics were shocking as well as the discovery that one serving size never sufficiently covers a baked potato. Counting condiments enabled me to see that I could fill the caloric needs of a small nation in one week with my salad dressing preferences alone. Let's face it, I had gained weight one tablespoon at a time. The proper consumption of condiments requires restraint, measurement, and the ability to walk away. I was in desperate need of retraining. A dollop is acceptable. A gravy boat is meant for all guests, not a party of one. I'm not suggesting that we ignore condiments. Indeed that world would be terribly dull. Is there any better complement to fish than a tangy lemon herb sauce? Creamy garlic butter should be a requirement on a warm hunk of sourdough. No, condiments are not to be vilified. But they are too good to resist and too caloric to ignore. Going into a condiment relationship blindly is waistline suicide. My solution—calculate and enjoy. Indulge in moderation and remember my revised mantra "Not every day's a hollandaise."

If you are wondering whether my fried clam epiphany curbed my consumption of tartar sauce, I'll have to let you know when I return to Connecticut (self-control in Pittsburgh is not a problem because you can't get fried whole belly clams in the 'Burgh). Twenty pounds lighter and still craving condiments, I will take my place in line at Lenny & Joe's Fish Tale, Captain's Galley, or Chowder Pot. But this time, I'm counting on moderation and the ability to clam up when I start to ask my husband for his portion of tartar sauce.

~Nancy Berk

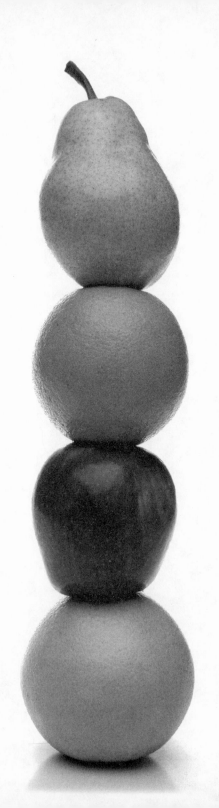

Chapter 10

Shaping the New You

Off the Beaten Path

*I will always focus on how far I have come
rather than how far I have to go.*

~Richard Simmons, The Book of Hope

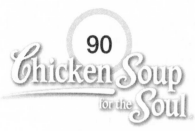
The Decaf Coffee Bar

Coffee smells like freshly ground heaven.
~Jessi Lane Adams

My mother was diagnosed with diabetes when I was nine. The adjustment from an operative pancreas to a non-functioning one changed my mother's life completely. A lifelong lover of sweet foods, my mother faced a constant battle against cravings for food she was not supposed to eat. At first she tried, so that nine-year-old me could enjoy cookies, ice cream, and candy at home, but it proved too much for her willpower. Boxes of cookies and pints of ice cream bought in the morning would be gone before I came home from school. She would be in tears from disappointment—over her own lack of control and for eating "my" sweets. I remember the day she announced that she couldn't trust herself to have ice cream and cookies in the house anymore.

From the first time I got an allowance, almost every cent was spent on Skittles, SweeTarts, Swedish Fish, Life Savers, and Sprees. I loved chocolate too, but the sugar rush provided by a handful of gummy bears was tough to beat. Once I remember grabbing a handful of candy corn from a bowl in a doctor's office, eating it on an empty stomach, and getting a sugar rush so powerful I had to lie down because the world was spinning so quickly. I never knew I could feel sick to my stomach and total bliss at the same moment.

You would think that the fear of getting diabetes myself would have curbed my behavior, but it didn't. Eating that much candy did only one thing. It made me fat. By high school, I was 30 pounds overweight. The funny fat girl in a group of cool girls, I wanted so badly to look like my pals. Finally in my senior year I crash-dieted and lost the weight, getting voted in my high school yearbook as "the girl who was most likely to disappear" since I had lost 30 pounds in two-and-a-half months.

By changing my eating habits I was able to stay in a healthy range for years — until I got pregnant with my first child. Despite trying to remain in control, my hormones were stacked against me, and after my daughter was born I held on to an extra 20 pounds. Atkins brought me back down before I became pregnant with my second child. After my son was born and the terrible twenty was back, the battle began again. I needed a long-term plan — one that did not include artery-clogging and crash diets.

Complicating the battle of the bulge were my two beautiful children, who, like most children, wanted dessert that was not fruit, peanut-butter chocolate-chip granola bars, not the boring oats-n-honey flavor, and a candy bar, lollipop, or piece of gum every time they saw one. Believing that denying my children might create even-worse sugar addicts, I have opted to have some sweet foods in the house and to limit the amount they can eat. At some point they will confront the ability to eat whatever they want, and hopefully helping them make smart choices now at home will help them make smart choices later by themselves.

To lose the 20 pounds that remained after my son was born I cut out bread, pasta, and desserts. Along with exercise, it took six months of chicken, fish, vegetables, fruit, water, and no dessert to lose it — a fine lifelong plan, except for the dessert. A lifetime of no dessert would never work for me. I had to come up with a solution. It came in the form of a decaf coffee bar.

Every night after we eat I give my kids some sort of dessert.

While they attack it like pit bulls, I open my decaf coffee cupboard and chose between regular, hazelnut or vanilla coffee beans. I grab my single-serve brewing filter and fill it full so that the coffee is strong and flavorful. Once brewed, I open the fridge and chose between milk, hazelnut-flavored milk, or vanilla-flavored milk. Finally I pick out a sweetener packet: pink, yellow, or green. Every night my options seem endless. Every combination tastes just a little bit different, takes about a half hour to drink, and the sweetness of it consistently curbs my craving. I love the fact that I get to make choices and my sweet tooth is tricked. I have managed to keep the extra weight off for five years and counting. Now, even when we got out to dinner I opt for decaf instead of dessert — unless, of course, they have bread pudding.

~Jennifer Quasha

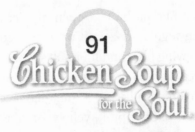

Just Eat

Life is really simple,
but we insist on making it complicated.
~Confucius

After years of spending hundreds (if not thousands) of dollars on diets, I finally figured out how to lose weight and stay fit. I just eat. I will never ever diet again. The sound of the word "diet" makes me shudder.

I wish I could say that I came to this epiphany on my own, but I didn't. A registered dietician named Dr. Maureen Latanick helped me. Actually I should say that she convinced me.

In January of 2008, I finally reached the breaking point. While I wasn't grossly obese, I needed to lose at least 20 pounds. I had been diagnosed as being insulin resistant, which is a precursor to diabetes. Frankly, going on another calorie or carb restricted diet seemed impossible to me.

Let me backtrack a few years. Like many young women of my time, I had a body image problem. My mother had allowed me to go on diet pills at the age of fifteen and so the yo-yo cycle of my food problems began.

I actually thought it was good not to eat. "Hunger is my friend," I would mumble to myself while my stomach growled uncontrollably. If I could keep my calories under 1,000 a day, I was a happy camper. To me, that meant that I was in control. I even had good food and bad food lists. Vegetables and proteins were good. Carbs were bad. Sugar was horrible.

My lists caused me to publicly restrict what I ate. But they also caused me to binge in the late evening when I felt deprived. Year after year this snowballed, but it wasn't until I visited Dr. Latanick that I actually came to terms with the fact that I wasn't a normal eater... in fact, I had (have) an eating disorder.

While I thought I was putting very few calories into my body, my "stand up never sit down at the table" eating definitely had plenty of calories. Enough to cause me to gain weight every time I went off a highly restrictive diet. And trust me, every time I went on a diet and lost a substantial amount of weight, I gained just as much back... if not more.

I had actually made my first visit to Dr. Latanick 10 years ago. When she told me I needed to eat, I didn't believe her. I saw her once or twice and then went back to Weight Watchers or Jenny Craig or something like that. Those programs are great for most people, but for me they are diets, and diets are bad for me.

This time when I went to see Dr. Latanick I was older, wiser, and tired of dieting with short-term results. Dr. Latanick convinced me to throw away my scales and begin to eat mindfully. She suggested a book or two which I read cover to cover.

The most meaningful thing that my dietician said to me was, "Look at it this way, if you only lose two pounds a month, in a year you will have lost 24 pounds that will stay off. In the process, you'll begin to learn how to use food like a normal person. Just eat."

"No restrictions at all?" I asked her.

"None," she said.

I'll never forget my first honest-to-goodness grilled cheese sandwich. I thought I'd died and gone to heaven. Up until this time, bread had been on my bad list, so grilled cheese sandwiches were unacceptable. Crazy as it sounds, a grilled cheese sandwich filled me with joy. Can you imagine that? Grilled cheese made me happy.

So did the corn, potatoes, and pasta. What I found was that when I allowed myself to eat, I didn't go crazy, I just ate. I mindfully and joyfully ate from all the food groups. I even allowed myself fast food without guilt when I was on the run.

From time to time I'd fall back to my old bad habits and Dr. Latanick would say, "A lapse isn't a relapse... just eat."

The pressure was off. The feeling of having to go on a diet was gone... especially since the scales were proving Dr. Latanick right.

Little by little I began to lose weight. There was never the thrill of a huge weight loss in one week like there had been on diets. There was however, the knowledge that with very little effort I could get slow but sure results.

Exercise has never been a problem for me. I ride my horse vigorously five days a week. Now, because I eat at regular intervals, my blood sugar is stable. I don't have highs and lows anymore. I am mindful of what I eat more often than not.

As the months have gone by the original excitement that I felt for eating has passed. In its place has come the confidence to know that I will never have to diet again. My guess is that I'll add a few years onto my already active life.

Food and eating are never going to be easy for me. Being mindful can be though. I've finally figured out that all I have to do is just eat. Imagine that.

~Jan Mader

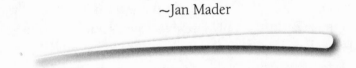

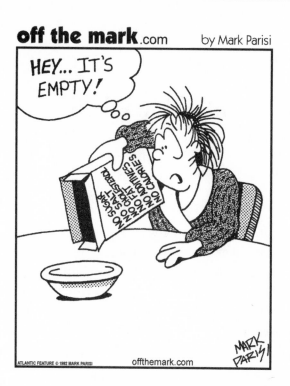

Reprinted by permission of Off the Mark
and Mark Parisi ©1997

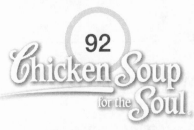

92

Arabian Abs

You wouldn't worry so much about what other people thought
if you realized how seldom they do.
~Eleanor Roosevelt

Y ou know those teenage girls who are able to gyrate and hip-hop like they were born knowing the right moves? I wasn't one of them. In fact, I spent many musical theatre dance classes watching those slender, toned girls execute perfect kick-ball-changes while I stumbled through the motions. I always assumed I just wasn't a dancer. Or an athlete. There's always that one kid in gym class who's half a lap behind everyone else, struggling to breathe without blacking out. That was me. I was an academic and a musician, and I was perfectly content to leave fitness to the real athletes.

It's interesting how university can change all of that. Struggling with the workload of first-year engineering, eating properly never once entered my mind. As exams rolled around, I quickly discovered that Kit Kat bars could soothe my frazzled nerves like nothing I had ever consumed before. As my jeans got tighter, however, my concern began to grow. I took to the university fitness centre with the best of intentions, but found myself intimidated by the regular varsity athletes who pumped iron and flexed in their Spandex. It felt as though even the professors were snickering at me as I sweated over the cross-trainer. My hyper-mobile patellae complicated matters and I soon found that 10 minutes on the cross-trainer would pinch my knees until I lost feeling.

Working out seemed pointless and frustrating, until one morning

I noticed a new poster on the change room bulletin board. A beautiful woman in a sparkling costume twirled across the glossy page, prompting me to take a closer look. Belly dancing classes! Get fit while being sexy. I was instantly attracted by the idea, but tentative too. Belly dancers were like exotic dancers, weren't they? Was this too brazen for me? More importantly, would I have to do a kick-ball-change?

It just so happened that my family sports club was offering beginner belly dancing classes the following fall. Being the trail-blazing, adventuresome — okay, total chicken — that I am, I begged my younger sister to come with me.

"Belly dancing? You're kidding, right?"

"It's like a fitness class. I really want to try it. Pleeease."

"I'm not showing my belly. I'm wearing baggy sweats."

"Fine! Come on. It'll be fuuunnn."

"You owe me."

We entered our first class with trepidation, almost wimping out completely and cancelling our registration. Gripping our courage tightly so that it couldn't make a dash for the door, we joined our classmates and instructor in a circle on the floor. Our teacher was a young, kind woman who asked us all why we chose to start belly dancing. I cited fitness as my reason, but as the beautiful, unfamiliar strains of Middle Eastern music filled the room, I realized I was going to get much more out of this class. Much to my surprise, I quickly found myself mimicking the instructor's movements without the same awkwardness that plagued me in musical theatre. Even arabesques, which at first glance seemed to be suspiciously ballet-related, didn't trip me up as previous lyrical dance movements had done. After that first class, I was hooked. Bitten by the belly dance bug, I rushed out to buy my own hot pink coin hip scarf and signed out every belly dance library book I could find.

It wasn't until a few months in that I first noticed the unthinkable. It took several minutes in front of a mirror to process what I was seeing, even as I flexed and twisted in different positions. Yes, they were really there — I had ab muscles! I could actually see the beginning of definition between the two major sides of my muscles. Pressing my hands into my stomach didn't feel like squishing marshmallows anymore. It was the first shred of evidence that I really could become fit, toned and thinner.

Entering the winter intermediate class challenged me to finally look at myself as a dancer. As our class repertoire of techniques increased, so did my confidence. I took pleasure in watching myself in the large dance mirror, always aiming for a front row spot instead of the back corner position I had claimed in high school. The addition of floating veils and more sparkling hip scarves touched my soul with all the allure and beauty of an Arabian Nights fantasy. I learned about the cultural significance of belly dance and the traditions behind what I used to incorrectly assume was an exotic, stripper dance. I got to spend more time with my sister, perform with her, and admire the graceful skills she was acquiring as well.

Somewhere under all the glitter and undulations, I learned to love my body. I gathered up the courage to try ballroom dancing, salsa dancing and even yoga. Most significant, however, was how comfortable I now felt entering a fitness centre. Instead of feeling judged, I realized that everyone else was too busy worrying about their own bodies to be concerned about mine. The people who once seemed intimidating were now my fellow comrades in fitness. For the first time in my life, I felt like I deserved to be there and I let myself really enjoy exercise.

Three years, 10 classes and two shows later, belly dancing has become the brightest spot in my week. For two precious hours a week, I forget about my lab deadlines and looming exams, and I focus completely on the partnership between my body and the music. I've stopped worrying about the way other people view my exercise habits or my body, because through all of it, I earned the best reward of all—my abs. Err, I mean, confidence.

~Emily Ann Marasco

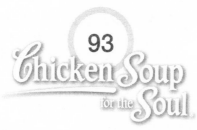

93

Face Workout

To exist is to change, to change is to mature,
to mature is to go on creating oneself endlessly.
~Henri L. Bergson

As I turned the corner, my daughter, Serrae yelled, "Mom, stop making those faces. One of my friends might see you."

"Yeah," said my son, Noah, as he slumped down in his seat. "They'll think you're crazy."

I continued puckering my lips in and out to the count of three. After completing five repetitions, I formed my mouth into the shape of an "O" while simultaneously pulling up my bottom jaw.

At the stoplight, I rhythmically rotated my head from left to right watching with each pivot to see if the light had changed. Out of the corner of my eye, I saw the lady in the car to my left staring at my swiveling neck.

When the light turned green, I pressed the accelerator and scrunched my forehead up and down. I then performed one of the most difficult exercises. I pressed my chin in and out 10 times while ignoring the slow burn traveling up the sides of my jaw.

"Mom, really. What's the purpose of this?" asked Noah.

Serrae, now disguised by my sunglasses and a baseball cap she found in the backseat, said, "Don't you think you exercise a little bit too much? Can you spell obsession?"

"Kids, what you don't understand is fitness doesn't start below the neck. We have 57 facial muscles and they need to be exercised just like the rest of our bodies. In order for those muscles to stay toned and tight, we have to increase the circulation to those areas. One of the best ways to accomplish this is by the exercises I'm doing. You want your mom to be healthy and look good, right?"

"I guess so."

"Whatever."

"I guess so" and "whatever" were hardly the responses I desired, but after a year of facial exercise, six days a week for 20 minutes, I had achieved the outcome intended and I am no longer mistaken for someone older than I really am.

There is beauty at every stage of life yet most of us want to look our age or younger—not older. When I look in the mirror, I genuinely embrace the fine lines, the slight downturn of my mouth, and the faint age spots because I know they are typical of my generation. Growing older is a blessing, but I want to look good for my age. I envision myself at seventy, eighty and ninety years old, strong and vibrant from head to toe. And yes, I'll still be traveling down the road—puckering up my face and perplexing the other drivers.

~Dwan Reed

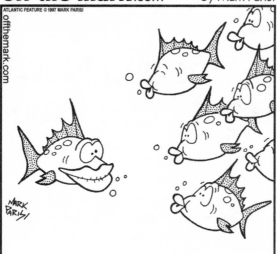

off the mark.com   by Mark Parisi

BRODERICK WOULD OFTEN ENTERTAIN
THE OTHERS BY MAKING PEOPLE LIPS

Reprinted by permission of Off the Mark
and Mark Parisi ©1992

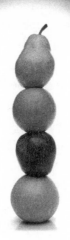

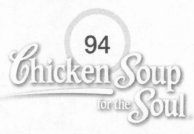

94

The Amazing Newborn Weight Loss Program

One way to get thin is to re-establish a purpose in life.
~Cyril Connolly

Quite by accident, I stumbled across an amazing and innovative method for losing weight. As a woman in my late 50s, I'm finding it difficult to overcome my slowing metabolism and my failing capacity for physical activity. The weight just keeps creeping up. But this unique weight loss program not only keeps you in shape, it has added perks.

It began with a simple gesture on my part to help my son after he and his wife returned to the States following a six-year stint in a foreign country. They were overwhelmed with the household upheaval, further complicated by the needs of two young children—a 22-month-old son and a four-week-old daughter. Wanting to help out anyway I could, I offered to take the newborn home with me for a short time to give her sleep-deprived mother a break while she sorted out the chaos at their new home.

Little did I know, I had signed up for an exercise and diet regime rivaled only by a military boot camp. I've been through this routine before, I told myself; I can handle it again. What I forgot was the fact that I was 35 years younger then. As the saying goes, "Mother Nature knows best." That's why she doesn't bestow these little packages on the "not so young anymore." But, in my eagerness to help, and my joy over having this tiny angel all to myself for a while, I bundled her up and headed for home — a mere five-hour drive away.

And that's when the unforeseen diet and exercise program began. Arriving home, I hit the ground running. First came the never-ending line of baby bottles to hand-wash, sterilize and fill with formula. After all, the baby was growing at an alarming rate and needed to eat every three hours around the clock.

I quickly settled into a routine where I snatched up the crying baby, ferried her off to the diaper changing station, and headed for the kitchen to warm a bottle. Next, I fed the ravenous, squirming little creature, and then bounced her on my knee to encourage that elusive bubble hiding in her tummy, waiting to disgorge the formula I had managed to coax through her perfect little lips.

In between these feeding crises, I continued to replenish the empty baby bottles in readiness for the next frantic cry. Then I faced the mountain of laundry these tiny people produce. Even though their diapers are disposable, they need clean sheets and blankets on their beds every day and at least two changes of clothing — more if the burping session isn't successful and the formula spews out onto their cute little footie pajamas.

By day three, I was bleary-eyed and dazed, but still thankful for each treasured moment I shared with my granddaughter. When I embarked upon my mission, I failed to realize the amount of energy it takes to jump out of bed three times every night and dash around all day to complete the never-ending baby-tending chores.

Sleep was becoming a highly prized commodity and food was an afterthought. One morning, while loading the dishwasher, I looked around for my cereal bowl, and realized, in my haste to feed and bathe the baby, then shower and get dressed before she awoke for the next round, I forgot to eat breakfast.

It was 11 o'clock, so I decided to treat myself to an early lunch. I prepared my favorite microwave pizza, practically drooling as I placed the steaming, spicy treat on the table. Unfortunately, my granddaughter began to scream before I took my first bite. An early lunch was on her agenda, as well.

Thirty minutes later, when I returned to my stone-cold pizza, it had lost its appeal. I tossed it in the fridge and scarfed down a handful of cashews and a few grapes. Lunch was over. It was time to tackle the laundry.

As the days passed, I realized that my new, active lifestyle, with little time to eat, was better for my waistline than my regular exercise routine. Bouncing a fussy baby for hours on end burned quite a few calories, and holding her at arm's length during the bouncing was better than weight training.

Towards the end of my babysitting assignment, I noticed that my slacks didn't seem quite as tight. I stepped on my bathroom scale and discovered I'd lost five pounds. This was no surprise, given the daily, 24-hour baby watch marathon I'd been through, but I certainly hadn't anticipated the weight loss benefit. This newborn baby-tending regimen was more effective than a "fat farm" and a heck of a lot cheaper.

My original intent was to help my son and his family through a trying time, but I was the one who was truly blessed. Not only did I manage to lose a few pounds, I will cherish the special time I shared with my granddaughter for the rest of my life.

When the final day of her visit arrived, my body weighed five pounds less, but my heart felt 10 pounds heavier. She had filled my life with joy and purpose during her brief stay, and I would miss her terribly.

The return trip seemed much too short, and I fought back tears as I parked the car at their curb. I thought nothing could ease the pain in my heart—until I saw the joy on her mother's face when she hugged her precious daughter.

It was a happy reunion for all of us. But I vowed right then and there to stay physically fit, because they might need my services again soon. Motivation is the key for weight loss success, and, for me, being able to keep pace with my grandkids is a powerful diet and exercise motivator. I'm now anxiously awaiting my next physical challenge: "The Amazing Two-Year-Old-Toddler Weight Loss Program."

~Gloria Hander Lyons

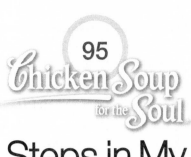

95

10,000 Steps in My Shoes

Make your feet your friend.
~J.M. Barrie

got a pedometer for Mother's Day and hadn't taken it out of the box. I had planned to walk all summer. Instead I told myself that I was getting plenty of exercise hanging around the shallow end of the town pool yakking with the other moms and eating fudgesicles (only 60 calories!) while the kids went off the high dive. Maybe the water just made me feel lighter. Anyhow, it was too hot to walk.

But then summer was over and it was a new school year. Along with my resolution to ban video games until next June, I also resolved to walk myself thin. Actually, I would have been happy to simply walk myself a little less fat. The brochure that came with the pedometer says that walking 10,000 steps a day will burn an extra 2,000-3,000 calories a week.

That's a lot of fudgesicles.

Sure, there are aerobic benefits to walking, too. But frankly, I don't really care what my left ventricle looks like — as long as my thighs are thin.

The American Council on Exercise ranks various professions and reveals that while mail carriers rack up 19,000 steps every day, secretaries take only an average of 4,327 steps at work, restaurant employees about 10,000 steps and custodians walk nearly 13,000 steps. I figured that my days most closely mirrored those of a custodian or a restaurant worker so I must have been logging the requisite 10,000 steps a day. Easy.

So one morning I clipped the pedometer to the waistband of my soon-to-be-a-size-smaller jeans and started counting steps. I walked downstairs and made coffee (13 steps) trotted back upstairs to wake up my son Lewis (17 steps), went down to the basement to get clean laundry (21 steps), and then upstairs again to tell Lew to hurry up (15 steps). After breakfast, I ran half a block chasing Lewis with the lunch he left on the kitchen counter (52 steps), dashed through the house looking for my car keys (37 steps), went grocery shopping and powered through the produce section, meat department and frozen food section (227 steps). At home I made six separate trips carrying bags from the car to the kitchen (47 steps) and put away the groceries (4 steps). Then I went upstairs to retrieve my glasses from the bedside table (15 steps) and settled down to work on the computer (0 steps). I also got up three times before lunch to let the dog out (18 steps). By noon, I had logged only a measly 466 steps. Only 9,534 steps to go.

The way I figured it, 10,000 steps is about five miles, which is approximately 80 minutes of walking. Eighty minutes! That's 40 minutes in each direction. I tell you, if I ever got 40 minutes away from my house I might never turn back.

I was tempted to cheat on the 10,000 steps by strapping the pedometer to my ankle and shaking my foot while I watched Oprah and ate fudgesicles, or clipping it on the dog's collar and letting him chase the squirrels through the backyards. Who, I wonder, other than the mailman, has time to walk 10,000 steps? Not me. No wonder my jeans were still snug.

I needed to find a way to walk more. So, after school, when I took Lewis and his friends to soccer practice, I also took my pedometer and my sneakers and, instead of sitting on the sidelines with the other moms or going home to start dinner, I walked around and around and around the field. During the hour of practice, I circled the field 12 times, bringing my grand total to 6,493 steps—more than halfway to my 10,000-step goal. Only 3,507 steps to go before bedtime. But hey, who's counting?

~Carol Band

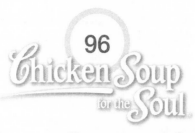

96

Taking Care of Me

The rewards for those who persevere
far exceed the pain that precedes the victory.
~Karen Bliss Livingston, elite road racer

The first time I stepped through the doors of a health club, I was thirteen. I was tagging along with my best friend after spending the night at her house. She had joined a local gym with her mom as a New Year's resolution to lose a few pounds. I distinctly remember an oval-shaped room, with a track running around the outside, and weight machines scattered throughout. Tracy headed for the track. I lay down in the carpeted area in the middle of the track and proceeded to go back to sleep.

That's what I thought of working out. In college, I joined a gym with a co-worker who was trying to "get toned," but every time I walked through the doors. I got the feeling that all eyes were on me. I imagined they were all wondering what "that skinny girl" was doing there. And to be honest, I've always felt lost in a gym, never sure if I was doing the right circuit, or using the machines correctly. Not to mention that I don't enjoy being watched by muscle-heads in wife-beaters to see if I can lift the 10-pound dumbbell over my head.

In my mid-20s, I started running with my husband, a New Year's resolution he had made to lose weight. And although I have a runner's frame, it did nothing to change my build or increase my lack of muscle.

All my life, I've been surrounded by friends and family who've tried to get in shape or lose a few pounds. All my life, the only times

I ever worked out, or walked into a gym, were for someone else. Not that I didn't have the metabolism of a speeding train, but in all honesty, I could have used the extra pounds many of them were carrying. Bird Legs, Bones, Bony Butt, Skeleton—I'd heard them all—especially throughout middle school and high school.

Then, at thirty-four, I found myself separated from my husband, a single parent of three kids, with a great deal of stress on my slight frame. I joined a local gym. Running, weight machines, recumbent bike, I did whatever I could to kick in those endorphins and alleviate some of my newfound stress. Still, over several months, I saw no difference in my frame, and although I felt better post-workout, I didn't feel any stronger or healthier.

During lunch one afternoon, I told my friend Kim about the gym I belonged to. "Oh, forget the gym," she said. "You ought to come to this boot camp I go to." Boot camp? I thought of a scene from *An Officer and a Gentleman*—a young Richard Gere hoisting a rifle over his head as he runs in place, while Louis Gossett, Jr. sprays ice cold water on his chest and face. "No thanks," I heard myself say. But, one look at her sculpted arms confirmed that this was a program that worked. I reluctantly agreed to attend a 90-minute Saturday session.

That Saturday morning was a turning point for me. After just 20 minutes, I was blinking back tears while I forced myself to finish just one more push-up on that muddy, grass hill. It was tough. Worse than tough. It was hell. Hill sprints, jumping jacks, sit-ups, push-ups, lunges, crawling uphill backwards on my hands and toes. More push-ups. More sit-ups. I went home, crawled into bed and woke up two hours later sure I had the stomach flu. Every muscle ached. Every breath hurt. But I was hooked. The next Saturday I showed up prepared for battle. By 9 a.m. it was already a typical humid St. Louis summer day. I was pushing myself, and stopped to take a long drink of water. And proceeded to throw it right back up.

It didn't stop me. It did teach me to come to boot camp fully hydrated, and to eat something healthy beforehand (as our instructor says, "Have a banana. They taste the same coming up."). And since I'd made it through two 90-minute sessions, I agreed to sign up for a full five-week program. Sixty minutes each, twice a week. Those first five weeks were slow. On the warm-up run, I was always at the end of the pack. Given a choice for the mid-session and post-session runs, I chose the "short run" with the other Newbies. I dropped to my knees for push-ups, and had to stop halfway through our two-minute sit-up drills just to give my stomach a break. But as my instructor says, "Exercise is either easy or effective. Never both. Which do you want?" Well, if I couldn't have both, I'd take effective. What was the point otherwise?

At the end of the five weeks, my instructor pulled me aside and asked about my eating habits. I admitted they weren't great, leaving out the details—skipped breakfasts, quick "lunches" of a candy bar and Coke standing at my desk, chips and salsa dinners when the kids were at their dad's. But I took his pages of notes and healthy diet plan samples and commenced reading. One thing he said stuck with me. "It doesn't make sense to work out as hard as you do, and then not eat right. The right mix of proteins, carbs and healthy fats," he reasoned, "will give you results that much quicker." And that made sense. Why push myself so hard during workouts only to go home and eat junk?

So, I got rid of the Coke and gave up fast food. Through my own actions, my kids are learning the value of exercise, nutrition and taking care of their bodies, too. When they have a stomachache, or are feeling tired, I say to them, "Tell me how you've taken care of yourself today." They have learned that the types of foods they put in their bodies have a direct effect on how they feel. And that exercise not only impacts how we look on the outside, but more importantly, changes how we feel on the inside. I've learned that this little body of mine is capable of much more than I ever gave it credit for.

It's been nine months since this bird-legged girl attended her first boot camp. It hasn't been easy, but it's definitely been effective. And for the first time in my life, I'm seeing the changes in the mirror. My arms are more muscular, my legs have shape, and my stomach muscles are well defined. It's a good feeling to know that at thirty-seven, I'm healthier than I was 15 years ago. Inside and out.

~Beth M. Wood

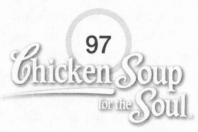

97

Surgery Isn't
the Easy Way Out

There are no shortcuts to any place worth going.
~Beverly Sills

I wanted a new start in life when I retired from the Army Nurse
Corps 20 years ago, so I moved my family from California to
Texas, bought a house, and started law school. All went well
except for one thing—in the process, I gained 70 pounds, going
from a size 10-12 to a 16W-18W in one year.

It wasn't supposed to happen that way. I'd had problems controlling my weight all my life, but I'd convinced myself that the
Army had ruined my metabolism by forcing me to weigh in every six
months for all those years. The consequences of being overweight
in the military included missing out on promotions and even being
asked to leave the service, so I managed to masquerade as a thin person at the weigh-ins by starving for a week or two beforehand, then
rushing home to stuff my face with pizza. Running and working out
helped a little, but my weight fluctuated by 10 to 15 pounds between
weigh-ins, and with age it became harder and harder to drop it. So,
I reasoned, retirement would allow me to stabilize at my "natural"
weight. Who knew that would be 212 pounds—and climbing?

I was raised to be a problem-solver, so I became my own favorite
project. I joined weight loss programs, lost a few pounds, then gained
them back. I tried walking, yoga, swimming, weight lifting, all with
dismal results. During this time, my husband's career required us

to move every year or two, so it seemed that every time I found a fitness routine I liked, we'd get the news we were moving across the country—again. I even tried medication and counseling after a physician told me that I must be depressed if I had to look at myself in the mirror every day! (He was fired for that remark, but his hurtful words stayed with me for years.)

When my older daughter announced her engagement, I panicked at the thought of shopping for a dress for the wedding. Plus size shops seem to cater to the "big-all-over" but there are few resources for women who are 5 feet tall and weigh 235 pounds. I settled for stretchy black pants and an ivory silk overblouse that I thought hid my fat pretty well—until I saw the wedding pictures. Next to the slender wedding party, I looked like something from another planet where short creatures with small heads and bowling-ball bodies were bred.

At fifty-five, I was squarely in the "morbidly obese" category, but I felt powerless to change. I was always hungry, and I fed that hunger with huge portions, lots of snacks, and sugar, sugar, sugar. I'd attended a 12-step program for overeaters for several years, and understood the concept of "stuffing" my feelings, but that didn't stop me eating like—and weighing the same as—a football linebacker.

Then I read an article about a woman who lost more than 100 pounds after praying for God to take away her overeating problem. That approach surely couldn't hurt, I thought, so I gave it a try—but nothing happened. I believed that God wanted people to be healthy and that He could intervene if we asked for help—I just didn't believe that He would want to help me. I was still hungry all the time and I was still fat, but I still prayed every day for a miracle—or at least just a couple of hours of feeling full.

Months later, I was still praying for a miracle every day when I happened to glance at a newsletter from my health insurer that I'd stuffed into a basket weeks before. Among the usual advice about flu shots and blood pressure checks, I noticed a brief paragraph about new benefits for weight loss surgery. I'd always thought of surgery as the easy way out and had never considered it for myself, so I threw the newsletter away, never thinking about it again until I heard myself at my next doctor's visit asking for a referral to a weight loss surgeon.

From that moment, I became obsessed with reading about bariatric surgery: books, magazines, on-line forums—I'd had no idea that so many resources existed. And I had plenty of time to read because it took eight months for my insurer to approve my first visit to a surgeon. After that, though, the process moved swiftly, and within a month I was being wheeled into the operating room for a laparoscopic gastric bypass operation.

I've learned since then that bariatric surgery is not the easy way out at all. Surgeons' guidelines vary, but most patients are restricted to a liquid diet for weeks before and after surgery. After a month or so, tiny meals of soft foods are allowed, but alcohol, sugary foods, and fizzy beverages are forbidden. Every bite must be chewed thoroughly, and the smallest miscalculation in texture or amount can cause digestive problems for hours.

Exercise was mandatory, too. I mostly walked and occasionally swam, but didn't do strength training as I should have. At first, I struggled to walk a couple of blocks, but after a few weeks I was able to add distance and speed.

And the weight dropped, which shocked me because I was convinced that I would be the only gastric bypass patient who actually gained weight. Unlike some patients who drop weight quickly, I lost 13 pounds the first week and 5-10 pounds each month after that. But I was losing inches, sometimes at a shocking rate. I looked at myself in the mirror one morning during the second month and realized that for the first time in many years, I had only one chin. There was a little wattle leftover, but during the night my double and triple chins had vanished.

And for the first time since I could remember, I no longer had that hunger that I'd never been able to satisfy. My itty bitty meals left me feeling full, and I even became something of a picky eater, passing up the high calorie foods on a buffet for lean meat and fruit.

Fifteen months after the surgery, I weigh 137 pounds and am just a few pounds from a normal weight for my height. I wear size

4-6 jeans, and medium tops. I have some saggy skin on my upper arms and thighs, so I'm not comfortable wearing shorts or sleeveless dresses, but I'm hoping that those areas will tighten up with exercise.

If not, I won't complain. At fifty-eight, I feel happier and more energetic than I did when I was forty. We moved to Hawaii six months ago, and every time I try something new—snorkeling, hiking on the volcano, exploring rain forests—I thank God for granting me the miracle of this new body, even if the way He made it happen wasn't quite what I'd expected.

~Marcy Brinkley

98

How I Clicked with Fitness

You don't have to run on a treadmill.
Find something you enjoy and just do it.
~David Snowdon

My sixth grade class was tested under the watchful eye of our physical education teacher as she held a clipboard and clicked a stopwatch. One of my classmates kneeled on my feet and held my ankles, while I rested on a mat, my knees bent like peaks. Click. Go! I led with the right elbow, then the left elbow, wobbling. Sit-ups counted only when both elbows touched both knees. My counting partner shouted out my score.

Click. On to push-ups. Click. Running. Click. Chin-ups. Several months later, our teacher presented some of my classmates a certificate signed by President Reagan and a round blue patch stitched with a gold eagle, the Presidential Physical Fitness Award. I never earned one. At eleven years old, I rationalized that this was okay because another set of test scores determined that I was reading at the high school level.

I didn't strive to be fit in high school either. By then, report cards were my interest. Physical fitness wasn't going to get me into college. If it was, my school would have offered it with an advanced placement (AP) option and my parents would have asked every night at dinner how I was doing in P.E.

In college, I avoided my grandmother and my aunt. They had started greeting me by commenting on how much weight I had gained, then bragging about how they never weighed more than 95 pounds. If I appeared hurt by their comments, they'd laugh and say that they were just making conversation. Over full plates at a holiday dinner, I confirmed that every woman in my family had a story about when Grandma told her she was fat. Today, when I thumb through old yearbooks and photos, my younger self doesn't look as bad as she felt.

After graduating from college, I traveled throughout Europe and Japan for my career, and by the time I was in my 30s, I stood 5'3" and weighed 200 pounds. With the guidance of the Weight Watchers program, I learned good eating habits such as portion control and smarter food choices. However, I took it a bit too far and lost 60 pounds in seven months. When Grandma saw me that spring, she gasped and couldn't say anything kind, so instead, she recalled when my behind was so big, it was "out to here."

Six years later, I regained 30 pounds during a stressful three-year work project. I worked at the office 70 hours a week, instead of working out, and my portion sizes grew, even though my choices weren't bad. I knew I could lose the weight again when the project ended earlier this year and without changing my diet or stepping into the gym, lost 15 pounds in three months. I can't explain this. Maybe the stress actually weighed 15 pounds? But soon enough, I reached a plateau and knew I would have to start working out, something I never enjoyed.

So I searched through WebMD for a new perspective. Many articles emphasized that heart disease was the biggest killer of women in the U.S. Forget dieting. I decided to watch my eating but really focus on getting my heart pumping. Exercise would no longer be tied to losing weight. Being fit and heart-healthy had become my new goal.

I looked up the Presidential Fitness Award program from grade school. Maybe their fitness tests could guide me or benchmark my progress? Presidentschallenge.org explained that the program had been expanded to include adults and seniors. The Presidential Active

Lifestyle Award program encourages adults to get at least 30 minutes of exercise five days a week. Click. Steps registered on a pedometer counted towards exercise credit. Click. If I exercised five days a week sometime in the next six to eight weeks, I would earn a certificate signed by President Obama and a blue square patch. The words next to the blue star read, "Sign me up!"

My apartment complex had just renovated its gym and I decided to return to the elliptical machine. These new machines were different, even equipped with a plug for my iPod and individual television screens. While working out, I tuned into The Food Network for the first time in years and learned that it was fun to watch Paula Deen fry food.

The log at presidentschallenge.org helped me plan and track my exercise. I began going to the gym regularly. I liked the fact that there was an online record of my efforts after I worked out. After 36 workouts, I earned the Presidential Active Lifestyle Award.

For me, working out had always been about right and wrong—right and wrong food, sizes, weight, and appearance. With the help of the presidentschallenge.org website, fitness is now an investment in my heart, in my future.

~Sherilyn Lee

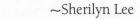

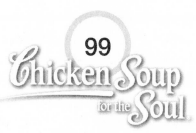

99

Granny-Size Helpings

Moderation is the silken string
running through the pearl chain of all virtues.
~Joseph Hall

"**I**'ll have another," I said to my friend after eating half a slice of her decadent cake. Christy already knew that I only indulged in halves, so she saved the other half for me in case I'd like more (sometimes I did if dieting wasn't the biggest issue at the moment).

Ever since I was a little tyke I would watch my grandmother, Margaret, serve everything in halves to her big family. There were nine kids and two adults in one house, and then some visiting grandkids, so it became a way of life for them to all have a small share of everything. Every time I went to her house we were served what she called "half portions," so no one went without. Cups of tea, cookies, cupcakes, cereal—everything—was halved, then quartered, or sliced paper thin so that everyone who wanted it could have some.

It was always the family joke when new guests were offered the infamous "granny-sized" portions. They would always be expecting a typical Thanksgiving-at-Grandma's giant-sized meal, and would instead find half of something on their plates. "There's usually more after everyone else is served," reassured the server, and the guests were usually understanding.

Even as the family size dwindled over the decades as the children grew and moved out, the rule of thumb was still "halves," mostly out of habit, but also because nothing went to waste. Grandma grew up in a big family, and was also a survivor of the Great Depression, so sharing small bits of everything was normal to her.

French chefs know that small portions are best because the eater will thoroughly enjoy just the first few bites of something anyway, and savor several different things instead of big portions like Americans do. The rest is simply "overindulgence," hence their familiar small portions of many courses in a formal meal.

And my very Irish grandmother already knew that secret from basic necessity.

When I need to watch my girlish figure I try to apply this simple "half of everything" principle, but always with a happy memory of my tiny grandmother, and her small platters of treats and drinks. I order a small size of something or automatically pack up half of the big meal or even an occasional dessert to save for later—or share. When I make a big meal it is with sharing in mind or to freeze it in small portions for easy-to-go, portion-controlled meals.

And now, visiting a friend who is also a very good baker, I don't even need to ask for a half slice anymore. She even calls it "granny-sized" because she knows me well and usually she eats the other half as we sip tea or wine and talk.

~Janice M. Wilson

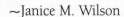

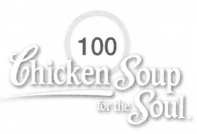

Keeping Busy

You are never too old to set another goal or to dream a new dream.

~C.S. Lewis

"Not this year," I answered my daughter. "Guess again!"

She studied me hard. "You didn't make a resolution to lose weight?"

"I said I didn't."

"Huh? That's your resolution every year."

"Look at me. Has it ever worked?"

She gave me the once over as I pirouetted in front of our refrigerator.

"I see your point," she admitted as she wiggled past me to open the fridge's door. "You don't buy healthy foods, Mom," she announced as she peered into the icebox.

"Like yogurt?"

"Yep."

"Seems to me I just tossed out a dozen containers someone stockpiled six months ago and never ate."

"They got pushed to the back. I didn't see them," she parried.

"And the Vitamin Water you had to have?"

"That stays good. Help yourself." She wandered off with some salsa to the pantry to claim an oversized bag of tortilla chips. I threw a withering glance at her choice for lunch. "You buy this stuff!"

"Your dad does."

I am 40 pounds overweight. And, I am never making a New

Year's resolution again about it. This past January I took a new tack. I limited my goals to four and losing weight's not one of them.

My premier objective is to learn how to dance. So, I take lessons at Fred Astaire once a week with a young Ukrainian instructor and also every Tuesday my husband and I attend group lessons at a local restaurant after hours. For those spans of time, I'm not eating; I'm moving and having fun.

My second aim is to walk daily. I have a gal pal who traipses around the neighborhood with me. Instead of jawboning on cell phones, we discuss politics, our kids, religion, gardening and local "gossip" as we perambulate. Again, I'm away from the pantry, moving and amusing myself.

My third goal's to organize my messes an hour a day. I don't mean mundane chores like daily dishes and laundry. I'm devoting 60 minutes per diem to long accrued piles, drawers of junk filled to the brim and crammed closets of stuff the PTA Thrift Shop would turn down. During this tidying time, my hands and mind are busy. I reach, grasp, and squat as I wrestle with decades of accumulated debris. No food involved in the process. Not a fun time but a sense of satisfaction surrounds me as I free up space.

My fourth pledge involves prayer. During this, I am stationary. Yet, it fixes my head, stabilizes my emotions, and gives me a renewed sense of purpose for all the tasks and diversions that lie ahead.

A month has passed since I resolved not to resolve to lose weight. Guess what? I've lost five pounds.

~Erika Hoffman

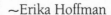

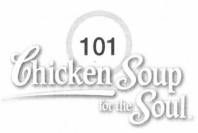

Three Easy Steps

No matter our age or condition,
there are still untapped possibilities within us
and new beauty waiting to be born.
~Dr. Dale Turner

had all but given up on dieting. Twenty years ago I invested in Nutrisystem and really lost a lot of weight, but I could not afford that now that I was no longer working. Times are hard, people are out of work and I guess you could say I fell into the habit of stress eating like so many others.

My crutch or "comfort food" as some would call it—was chocolate brownies with thick chocolate frosting. I started out with one brownie a week. It was my special treat. Soon that treat increased to one every other day, then one per day, then two per day—then I just do not know what happened.

I could actually sit down and eat a tray of brownies all by myself. And a big jug of milk to go with it. My clothes started fitting snugly—but I was approaching my mid-50s and didn't know many other women my age fretting over their weight all that much, so I didn't either. That is because I had been put on long-term disability by my employer, with fibromyalgia, systemic lupus, discoid lupus, chronic fatigue, high blood pressure, elevated sugar factor, etc.

I tried to join Weight Watchers but I did not qualify because of the elevated sugar factor. I couldn't afford Nutrisystem and so I became depressed on top of everything else. At this point I weighed almost 200 pounds.

One day I was getting my hair done and started talking to the girl who does my hair. She had lost 86 pounds in the last year. I asked her how she did it. She said she had her stomach stapled. She told me that her weight had been affecting her health and her doctor had prescribed a gastric bypass for health reasons. Her insurance company paid for it. I knew my problem was not the same as hers. Mine had to do with just plain overeating. My hairdresser told me to do three things and she guaranteed I would lose the weight faster than with any diet ever put on the market.

Number 1. Thank God for the body you have — every night and every day. Visualize the size you want to be and thank God for it. I wanted to be a size 10. I thanked God for making me a perfect size 10.

Number 2. Eat anything you want — but eat off a cake plate, not a dinner plate. This is for breakfast, lunch and dinner. Eat slowly, appreciating every bite. No second helpings. Drink lots of water.

Number 3. Get out and walk, walk, walk. I walk the local mall on Monday, Wednesday and Friday. It has two levels. By the time I have walked both levels I have broken a sweat.

I have done this faithfully for seven months and have lost 33 pounds, and I have gone from a size 20 to a size 12.

This has become a way of life for me and I don't believe I will ever go back to eating the way I did before. I feel so much better. My grocery bill is much lower. I have not had to invest in a diet program and my blood pressure is under control, my blood sugar is normal, my lupus is in remission and life is good.

~Linda J. Rivers

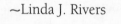

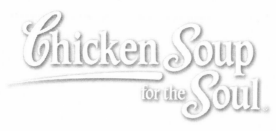

Meet Our Contributors

Debbie Acklin believes that having realistic expectations is just another way of setting limitations on herself. She travels as much as possible and is looking forward to her next adventure with her husband Perry and her two grown children, Amy and Greg. Contact her via e-mail at d_acklin@hotmail.com.

Lynne Albers earned an Elementary Education degree from Fort Hays State University in Hays, KS, and taught for several years before raising their now-grown children, Jennifer and Wade. Lynne and her husband Bob enjoy exploring the picturesque New Mexico landscape with their dog, Phoebe. You may e-mail her at lynnealbers@yahoo.com.

Christopher Allen writes Southern humor, both fiction and non-fiction. His work has been anthologized in *Chicken Soup for the Soul* and *Gathering: Writers of Williamson County* as well as in the e-zines *Metazen* and *Every Day Fiction*, among others. He writes about his travels at www.imustbeoff.blogspot.com.

Monica A. Andermann lives on Long Island with her husband/proofreader Bill and their cat Charley. When she is not writing, she enjoys reading and spending time with friends and family. In addition to two previous *Chicken Soup for the Soul* credits, her poetry and essays have been widely published both online and in print.

Jennifer Azantian received her Bachelor of Science, with honors, from the University of California, San Diego in 2010. She plans to pursue a Ph.D. in child psychology. Jennifer is also an author of several short stories and novels. Information about her fantastical tales can be found on her website: www.theeternallink.com.

Suzanne Baginskie has published many short stories, articles and poems and appears in eight other *Chicken Soup for the Soul* books. Retirement allows her to spend her free time writing and she is currently penning a legal thriller novel. She teaches a creative writing course at her local college. Visit Suzanne at http://mysite.verizon.net/resv10om.

Carol Band is an award-winning humor writer whose work appears in publications nationwide. In her spare time, she raises champion dust bunnies and kills houseplants. To read more, visit her website at www.carolband.com or her blog at www.carolband.wordpress.com.

Nancy Berk, Ph.D. is a psychologist, author (*Secrets of a Bar Mitzvah Mom*), and comic. She has written for More.com, Weight Watchers, and *Chicken Soup for the Soul*. Her second book, a humorous survival guide for parents of college applicants, will be available in 2011. Contact her at www.nancyberk.com.

Jan Bono taught school for 30 years on the Long Beach peninsula in southwest Washington State. She now works as a life coach, writing coach, Law of Attraction presenter, and freelance writer, with numerous articles and several books to her credit. Check out her blog at: www.daybreak-solutions.com/blog.

Ginny Dent Brant is an educator, counselor, writer, soloist, Christian speaker and Bible teacher who resides with her husband Alton in Clemson/Seneca, SC. Her first book, *Finding True Freedom: From the White House to the World*, will be released in the summer of 2010. Please e-mail her at ginnybrant@msn.com.

Marcy Brinkley, RN, JD, moved with her husband to Hawaii in 2009 where they enjoy snorkeling, hiking, and camping with their dogs.

They hope to visit frequently with the kids and grandkids back on the mainland. Marcy is working on an inspirational romance novel. Please contact her at marbrink@aol.com.

Douglas M. Brown has been writing since he was twelve years old. He has been published in several religious magazines, in *Chicken Soup for the Latter-day Saint Soul* and *Chicken Soup for the New Mom's Soul*. He lives in West Jordan, UT. You may contact Doug via e-mail at d8snraysons@yahoo.com.

John P. Buentello is the author of numerous short stories, essays, biographies, the novel *Reproduction Rights* and the short story collection *Binary Tales*. Currently he is at work on a new novel and a collection of connected short stories. Contact him at jakkhakk@yahoo.com.

Debbie Cannizzaro received her Bachelor of Arts in Elementary Education from the University of New Orleans. She is the author and illustrator of *We Live in Mandeville*. When Debbie isn't reading and writing, she enjoys making wheel-thrown pottery in her home studio. She and her husband Sal have three children: Nicole, Louis and Joseph.

A popular speaker at conferences and retreats, **Emily Chase** is the author of six books, including *Why Say No When My Hormones Say Go?* and *Help! My Family's Messed Up*. Visit her at emilychase.com to learn more about her writing and her speaking schedule.

Jeri Chrysong wakes up every morning grateful for her miracle, losing 170 pounds without surgery or drugs. She enjoys long walks along the beach with her pug, Mabel. Jeri also enjoys writing, photography, traveling and being a grandma. Visit Jeri's Remarkable Weight Loss Blog at http://jchrysong.wordpress.com.

Harriet Cooper is a freelance writer, editor and language instructor. She specializes in writing creative nonfiction, humor and often writes about health, exercise, diet, cats, family and the environment.

A frequent contributor to *Chicken Soup for the Soul*, her work has also appeared in newspapers, magazines, newsletters, anthologies, websites and radio.

Kyle Therese Cranston currently works as a content specialist/copywriter in Boston where she also teaches creative writing part-time at the Boston Center for Adult Education. In her spare time, Kyle enjoys writing, hanging out at bookstores, dancing to 80s music, and spending time with friends.

Ruth Douillette is an essayist and a photographer. She reviews books for various venues, including the Internet Review of Books where she is Associate Editor. After a day at her laptop, she heads to the gym — some days more enthusiastically than others. Come visit her blog Upstream and Down. http://upstreamanddown.blogspot.com.

Drema Sizemore Drudge is a 2008 graduate of Manchester College and is currently in the MFA program at Spalding University. She is an instructor with the Learn More Center in North Manchester, Indiana, where she and her husband Barry also reside. She is currently writing her first novel.

Melissa Face lives in Virginia with her husband and dog. She teaches, writes, and tries to squeeze into size 10 jeans. E-mail Melissa at writermsface@yahoo.com.

Patricia Fish is a blogger who writes book, movie, restaurant and TV reviews. She is a Backyard Wildlife Habitat trainer and her yard is certified as a Backyard Wildlife Habitat by the National Wildlife Federation. Pat loves to garden and loves the bird fellows. Her blog is http://patfish.blogspot.com.

Peggy Frezon writes a twice-monthly column "5 Things About Pets" and has stories in *The Ultimate Dog Lover*, *Miracles and Animals*, and others. She's a contributing writer for *Guidepost* magazine. Her first book, *Losing it With My Dog*, is about dieting with her chubby spaniel. Visit her blog: Peggy's Pet Place (peggyfrezon.blogspot.com) Twitter: @ peggyfrezon.

Sally Schwartz Friedman, a frequent contributor to the *Chicken Soup for the Soul* series, writes personal essays for national and regional publications including *The New York Times, AARP The Magazine* and *The Philadelphia Inquirer*. She is married to a retired judge, the mother of three daughters and a grandmother of seven. E-mail her at pinegander@aol.com.

Bracha Goetz is the Harvard-educated author of 12 children's books, including *The Happiness Box* and *The Invisible Book*. She also coordinates a Jewish Big Brother Big Sister Program in Baltimore, MD. Bracha can be reached at bgoetzster@gmail.com. Her story was reprinted with permission from www.TheJewishWoman.org, a project of www.Chabad.org.

Elaine K. Green is a native New Orleanian. She loves tennis, reading, and writing flash fiction. You may e-mail her at ekgreen@hotmail.com.

Judy Gruen is the author of three award-winning humor books, including *The Women's Daily Irony Supplement*. Her essays have appeared in the *New York Daily News, Chicago Tribune, The Boston Globe, Ladies' Home Journal*, and dozens of other media outlets. Enjoy more of her work at judygruen.com.

Alison Gunn is a writer who lives in Victoria with her husband and two daughters. She was previously published in *Chicken Soup for the Girl's Soul*. E-mail Alison at alisheehan@yahoo.com or visit her blog at http://cautiousmum.wordpress.com.

Lucinda Gunnin is a writer and mini-storage manager living in Illinois. She was diagnosed with multiple sclerosis in 2005, four years after suffering symptoms. The symptoms disappeared with her change in diet. Lucinda has also been published in *Elements of Time* and *Elements of the Soul* from Twin Trinity Media.

Christina Marie Harris is a 20-something Jersey Shore Girl with a sharp tongue and an even sharper pen. A freelance writer by trade, she also works at Precision Garage Doors. (www.precisiongaragedoorsnj. com). She is also published in *Chicken Soup for the Soul: Devotional Stories for Women*. Contact her via e-mail at WordsByChristina@gmail.com.

Rebecca Hill lost 40 pounds with Weight Watchers and is now a Circuit Coach at Curves in Marina del Rey, CA. She remains a huge fan of her former boss, Kiana Tom, and encourages everyone to check out Kiana's websites for fantastic health and fitness tips! www. fitmomtv.com and www.kiana.com.

Erika Hoffman has published inspirational, humorous, and travel pieces for an array of magazines and anthologies. She can be reached via e-mail at bhoffman@nc.rr.com.

Theresa Hupp is a prize-winning author of novels, short stories, essays and poetry. She is also an attorney, mediator and human resources executive. Theresa is a member of the Kansas City Writers Group and the Oklahoma Writers' Federation, Inc. She can be reached via e-mail at MTHupp@gmail.com.

Since 1995, **Rabbi Mitchell M. Hurvitz** ("Rabbi Mitch") has served as the spiritual leader for Temple Sholom of Greenwich, CT. A well-published author of articles and columns, he also co-authored Facts on File's *Encyclopedia of Judaism*. Please subscribe to his weekly teachings by contacting him directly at rabbimitch@templesholom.com.

Kimberly Hutmacher is the author of eight books for children, including a picture book titled *Paws, Claws, Hands and Feet*. Besides spending time with her family and writing, she also loves to exercise!

Learn more about Kimberly and read her book reviews at http://wildaboutnaturewriters.blogspot.com.

Peggy James lives in Durham, NC, where you can often see her out walking. She has walked six half marathons so far, and hopes to one day walk a full marathon.

Christine Junge is a writer and editor living outside of Boston, MA, with her husband and many pets. She teaches writing throughout the Boston area. Christine has an MFA in creative writing from Lesley University. She would love to hear from readers via her blog (www.writerbug.blogspot.com) or e-mail (christinejunge@hotmail.com).

Ron Kaiser, Jr. lives in New Hampshire with his beautiful and charming wife Meghan, and their three small dogs. He is currently seeking representation for a book of short stories, a novel, and the amazing true story of his father, who just so happens to be his hero. E-mail him at kilgore.trout1922@gmail.com.

Shannon Kaiser received her BA in Journalism and Communication from the University of Oregon. She is passionate about travel, writing and endurance sports, and just completed her first half Ironman triathlon. She lives in Oregon with her favorite jogging buddy, her dog Tucker. Contact her at www.travelpod.com/syndication/rss/shannonkaiser or Shannon.kaiser@mac.com.

Elizabeth Kelly is a freelance magazine writer living in Knoxville, TN with her fiancé, teenage daughter, five cats, two fire toads and a dwarf hamster. Her obsessions include Crock-Pots and P.G. Wodehouse novels. Contact her via e-mail at ekellywrites@gmail.com.

Nancy B. Kennedy has published two Bible story and science activity books for children: *Make It, Shake It, Mix It Up* and *Even the Sound Waves Obey Him* (Concordia Publishing House). She writes books, articles and essays, and blogs about other people's weight loss success. Visit her website at www.nancybkennedy.com.

April Knight is an artist and freelance writer. She lives in Washington. She recently spent six months in Australia where she rode a camel 50 miles in the Outback. She has just finished writing a series of five romance novels. Contact her at moonlightlady1@hotmail.com.

Terri Knight has a degree in psychology, substitute teaches and has several pieces published. "Forward" won the 2007 Fiction Contest at Edison College. Later, *St Anthony's Messenger* published it. She finished her first romance novel, *Finding Home*, and is starting her next one, *Look Who's Dating a Soap Star*.

Kathleen Kohler writes for magazines and anthologies on a variety of topics. She lives with her husband in the Pacific Northwest. Besides writing, she enjoys gardening, travel, relaxing at the beach, reading, and watercolor painting. To read more of her published work, visit www.kathleenkohler.com.

Nancy Julien Kopp draws from life experiences for essays, stories, poems, and articles. Her work is in nine *Chicken Soup for the Soul* books, other anthologies, magazines, newspapers, and e-zines. A former teacher, she still enjoys teaching through the written word. She blogs at www.writergrannysworld.blogspot.com. E-mail her at kopp@networksplus.net.

As a hobby, **Heidi Krumenauer** has published eight books, more than 1,200 articles, and has contributed chapters to more than a dozen book projects. Her career, however, is in upper management with an insurance company in Madison, WI. Heidi is a 1991 graduate of the University of Wisconsin-Platteville.

Annie Kuhn received a BA in art from Macalester College and an MFA in Writing for Children and Young Adults from Vermont College. She currently teaches English at Eastern Maine Community College and works for a children's bookstore. Annie loves travel, art, history, and eating out! Contact Annie via e-mail at anniekuhncreates@gmail.com.

Jennifer Leckstrom works in public relations. She earned a Bachelor of Science degree in communication at The University of the Arts in Philadelphia. She resides in the Pocono Mountains of Pennsylvania with her husband and two stepchildren. She enjoys traveling and sipping good bourbon. Please contact her via e-mail at jleckstrom@gmail.com.

Sherilyn Lee holds a Master of Fine Arts (MFA) degree in Creative Nonfiction from Antioch University Los Angeles. Her writing has been published by *Prism Review*, *Kauai Backstory*, *Quiet Mountain Essays* and other journals. She may be contacted via e-mail at sherilynlee@ sherilynlee.com or on Twitter @sherilynwrites.

Gloria Hander Lyons has channeled 30 years of training and hands-on experience in the areas of art, interior decorating, crafting and event planning into writing creative how-to books, fun cookbooks and humorous slice-of-life short stories. Visit her website to read about them all: www.BlueSagePress.com.

Jan Mader lives in Columbus, OH with her husband Chuck. She has a passion for animals and animal rescue. Jan loves spending time with her grandchildren and riding her horse Tango. Jan is the author of numerous children's books. She has blogs for writers and animal lovers at http:// ignitetowrite.blogspot.com and http://animaltalk4u.blogspot.com.

Emily Ann Marasco is finishing a degree in computer engineering and a minor in music at the University of Calgary. In her time outside of the lab, she enjoys playing her oboe, reading, and belly dancing. Emily is a student columnist for APEGGA, and is working on a fantasy novel.

Mimi Marie is a mother of two boys and works part-time in the medical field. Mimi enjoys yoga, fishing, and her volunteer work with

Prison Ministry. She plans to continue writing inspirational articles and sharing the hope available through Christ Jesus.

David Martin's humor and political satire have appeared in many publications including *The New York Times*, the *Chicago Tribune* and the *Smithsonian Magazine*. His humor collection, *My Friend W*, was published in 2005 by Arriviste Press. David lives in Ottawa, Canada with his wife Cheryl and his daughter Sarah.

Toni L. Martin is a programmer-analyst by day and a group leader for the Florida Writers Association by night. Both are sedentary jobs. Her personal trainer, a 10-pound Italian Greyhound, does his best to keep her in shape in her spare time.

Beth (Waterkotte) Molinaro received her Bachelor of Science from Indiana University of Pennsylvania in 1981. She lives in New Milford, CT and enjoys spending time with her husband Anthony and their children, Zach and Annie. She describes her writing as "quick-witted & warm-hearted." Please e-mail her at bam1013@charter.net.

Lisa Coll Nicolaou graduated from Yale University. She is a middle school teacher and an aspiring writer. She still tries to get to the gym every morning. Lisa appreciates a good laugh and the support of her friends and family. Read more at laughwithlisa.blogspot.com or e-mail her at lcn0404@aol.com.

Linda O'Connell is an award-winning writer, poet and teacher in St. Louis, MO. Her essays appear in 11 *Chicken Soup for the Soul* books, numerous anthologies, literary and mainstream publications. Her idea of happiness is strolling hand in hand with her husband on a warm summer's eve. Contact her via e-mail at billin7@yahoo.com or http://lindaoconnell.blogspot.com.

Caroline Overlund-Reid grew up in Oregon and attended St. Olaf College in Northfield, MN. She is currently "retired" but works two days a week in her daughter's consulting business. She enjoys writing, water colors, volunteer activities, her grandchildren, friends and family. She has been writing most of her life. She can be reached via e-mail at creid@bak.rr.com.

Mark Parisi's "off the mark" comic, syndicated since 1987, is distributed by United Media. He won the National Cartoonists Society's award for Best Newspaper Panel in 2009. His humor also graces greeting cards, T-shirts, calendars, magazines, newsletters and books. See www.offthemark.com. Lynn is his wife/business partner. Daughter Jen contributes inspiration, as do three cats, one dog, a frog and an unknown number of koi.

Faith Paulsen's writing has appeared in *Literary Mama*, *Wild River Review*, *A Cup of Comfort for Parents of Children with Special Needs* and *A Cup of Comfort for Mothers*. Dennis Chipollini is a motivational speaker, personal trainer, and founder of Generation Hope.

Laurie Penner works full-time in computer assisted design (CAD). When she's not helping her husband David build their house, she enjoys gardening, quilting, rock hunting, and spending time with their four grandchildren. Laurie plans to expand her writing career in her retirement years. Please e-mail her at writer7laurie@gmail.com.

Saralee Perel, an award-winning columnist and novelist, is honored to be a multiple contributor to *Chicken Soup for the Soul*. Saralee is agented for her book about her dog who became her caregiver after Saralee suffered a spinal cord injury, and her cat who kept her sane. Contact her via e-mail at her sperel@saraleeperel.com or through her website www.saraleeperel.com.

Lori Phillips lives in Southern California with her husband and children. Her husband plans to move the family into a one-story home so he can enjoy cheesecake once again. You can e-mail her at hope037@ hotmail.com.

Sheri Plucker is a freelance writer who has published articles and children's books on Down syndrome including *Me, Hailey!* She has a B.A. in Recreation Management from Eastern Washington University. She is inspired by her three children. Her youngest, Hailey, has Down syndrome. The family resides in Snohomish, WA. Contact her at splucker@msn.com.

Jeanne-Marie Poulin earned an Associate of Arts degree from Capital Community-Technical College in 1996. She is currently employed at a local elementary school and lives in Glastonbury, CT with her husband, daughter and Schnauzer. She also has a grown daughter and two grandchildren. Jeanne-Marie loves reading, writing, photography and traveling.

Felice Prager has accumulated hundreds of local, national, and international credits in print and on the Internet. Many of her essays have been included in popular anthology series including several *Chicken Soup for the Soul* volumes. She is the author of *Quiz It: Arizona*—www. QuizItArizona.com. Contact her via e-mail at felprager@cox.net.

Jennifer Quasha is a freelance writer and editor who loves reading, and writing for, *Chicken Soup for the Soul* books. You can check out her website at www.jenniferquasha.com, and see some of what she's been doing since she went freelance in 1998.

Dwan Reed, a licensed Master of Social Work, and preacher's wife, resides in Houston, TX. She spends her time as a professional public speaker, freelance writer, prison evangelist, and real estate agent. She can be contacted at dwanbooks@yahoo.com.

Few topics make **Nancy Higgins Reese** as enthusiastic as health and positive body image. Check out her blog at www.fatgirlskinnygirl. wordpress.com. Nancy has written several children's books. In her spare time, Nancy enjoys singing, skiing, and spending time with her family.

Natalie June Reilly is a freelance writer and a single "football" mom of two extraordinary teenage boys. She is also the author of the children's book, *My Stick Family: Helping Children Cope with Divorce*. If she hasn't escaped with her family to the beach, Natalie can be reached via e-mail at natalie@themeanmom.com.

Linda J. Rivers is a California native, now residing in the state of Minnesota with her husband Ernie, a retired military officer with the United States Army, and eleven-year-old daughter, Kira. She began her writing career in 1980 as a weekly columnist for the *Statesman Journal* newspaper in Salem, OR.

Amanda Romaniello graduated from Syracuse University in 2010. This is her second story in a *Chicken Soup for the Soul* book. Amanda loves to write, read, bake and spin. She writes about her love life in the blog "Fool for Love." Contact her at amanda.romaniello@gmail.com.

Jo Russell is an inspirational writer living in northeast Arizona. She retired as a reading teacher five years ago and now sells home décor. Jo has a number of books in the making including a humorous women's devotional titled *Which Button Do You Push to Get God to Come Out?*

Linda Sabourin lives in Oklahoma. She enjoys reading, writing short stories and poetry, watching football and drag racing, and tinkering with old computers. She has seven cats and a boyfriend who has five... and often wonders what the future will bring... kittens, perhaps?

Deborah Shouse is a speaker, writer and editor. Her writing has appeared in *Reader's Digest*, *Newsweek*, and *Spirituality & Health*. She is donating all proceeds from her book *Love in the Land of Dementia: Finding Hope in the Caregiver's Journey* to Alzheimer's programs and research. Visit her website at www.thecreativityconnection.com.

A career development professional, **Fran Signorino** is a career staff writer on Examiner and Factoidz; she also writes under the name,

Marie Coppola. Having received her BS degree with honors in 1993, she was a human resource administrator until she retired to the beach and sun in South Carolina. You can e-mail her at mcopp@ymail.com.

Tulika Singh is a freelance writer and copyeditor. She has earlier worked with leading Indian dailies including *Hindustan Times* and *The Times of India*. She currently divides her time between the two loves of her life—writing and her four-year-old twins. Please e-mail her at tulika20@hotmail.com.

Lynetta Smith is a homeschooling mom and freelance writer. She lives with her husband and daughters in Nashville, TN.

Peter D. Springberg, MD is a retired Air Force nephrologist and former medical center commander now living in northern Colorado. He's been a story teller for nearly 40 years, a writer for six. His twice-weekly blog on diet/lifestyle issues is embedded in his website http://PeterDSpringbergMDFACP.com.

Johnna Stein wears many hats: reading therapist, mother of two wonderful teenagers, freelance writer, women's program director at her church and wife to her Prince Charming. Her non-fiction stories have appeared in children, teen and adult magazines. She is currently working on finding a home for her humorous middle grade novel.

Sandra Stevens was raised in Florida and lives in Seattle where she is currently working on a novel. She is inspired by family, good food, warm friends and great literature.

Kim Stokely received her undergraduate and master's degrees in drama. She has toured churches throughout the country in a one-person musical about women in the Bible. She lives in Nebraska with her husband and an assortment of creatures including two teenagers and two dogs. Please visit her at kimstokely.com.

Sharon A. Struth is a graduate of Marist College. She lives in Bethel, CT with her husband and two teenage daughters. Her work can also be seen in *Chicken Soup for the Soul: My Resolution*, *Chicken Soup for the Soul: Power Moms*, *Sasee Magazine*, *A Cup of Comfort for New Mothers*, and WritersWeekly.com.

Tsgoyna Tanzman's career spans from belly dancer, to speech pathologist, to fitness trainer, to memoir teacher. Writing is her "therapy" for raising her adolescent daughter. Published in three *Chicken Soup for the Soul* books, her essays and poems can be read online at More.com, motheringmagazine.com, and *The Orange County Register*. E-mail her at tnzmn@cox.net.

B.J. Taylor loves how she feels and how she looks, which keeps her motivated to make wise choices. She is an award-winning author whose work has appeared in *Guideposts* and many *Chicken Soup for the Soul* books. She has a wonderful husband, four children and two grandsons. You can reach B.J. at www.bjtayloronline.com.

Elaine Togneri is published in non-fiction, short fiction and poetry. She is the founder and a past president of the Sisters in Crime — Central Jersey chapter, and the editor of *Crime Scene: New Jersey*. Elaine holds an MA in English from Rutgers Graduate School. Visit her website at sites.google.com/site/elainetogneri.

Thurmeka Ward received her Bachelors of Art from St. John's University and is currently obtaining her Masters in General and Special Education. She enjoys writing, singing, and working with children. She plans to continue writing in various areas. Please e-mail her at tward69@gmail.com.

Stefanie Wass's essays have been published in *The Los Angeles Times*, *Seattle Times*, *Christian Science Monitor*, *Akron Beacon Journal*, *Akron Life and Leisure*, *Cleveland Magazine*, *A Cup of Comfort for Mothers*, *A*

Cup of Comfort for a Better World, and seven *Chicken Soup for the Soul* anthologies. Visit her website at www.stefaniewass.com.

Bill Wetterman managed and trained some of the finest professional search consultants in the country before retiring from Wolters Search Group. He is a member of several professional writers' organizations. Bill writes both non-fiction and fiction short stories and novels. You can reach Bill via e-mail at bwetterman@cox.net.

Janice M. Wilson has been a writer since her early teens. She is finishing her second novel, writes poetry, short stories, and founded a writers' group based in southern New Jersey, where she lives with her daughter. She also enjoys the outdoors, reading, and cooking. E-mail Janice at beachladynj@yahoo.com.

Beth M. Wood lives in St. Louis with her three beautiful children and one three-legged Boxer. She is a marketing professional by trade, a writer by choice, a devout reader and semi-fanatic editor who will occasionally sneak a red Sharpie into restaurants to correct glaring, grammatical errors on the menu.

Joanna G. Wright is a freelance writer from Indianapolis, IN, where she resides with her husband and two daughters. She enjoys reading, gardening, drawing and quilting.

Susan Kimmel Wright lives in a western Pennsylvania farmhouse with her husband and an ever-changing assortment of animals and adult children. She has authored three children's mystery novels and many *Chicken Soup for the Soul* stories. Contact her at floatingagainstthecurrent.blogspot.com.

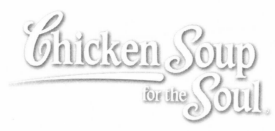

Meet Our Authors

Jack Canfield is the co-creator of the *Chicken Soup for the Soul* series, which *Time* magazine has called "the publishing phenomenon of the decade." Jack is also the co-author of many other bestselling books.

Jack is the CEO of the Canfield Training Group in Santa Barbara, California, and founder of the Foundation for Self-Esteem in Culver City, California. He has conducted intensive personal and professional development seminars on the principles of success for more than a million people in twenty-three countries, has spoken to hundreds of thousands of people at more than 1,000 corporations, universities, professional conferences and conventions, and has been seen by millions more on national television shows.

Jack has received many awards and honors, including three honorary doctorates and a Guinness World Records Certificate for having seven books from the *Chicken Soup for the Soul* series appearing on the New York Times bestseller list on May 24, 1998.

You can reach Jack at www.jackcanfield.com.

Mark Victor Hansen is the co-founder of Chicken Soup for the Soul, along with Jack Canfield. He is a sought-after keynote speaker, bestselling author, and marketing maven. Mark's powerful messages of possibility, opportunity, and action have created powerful change in thousands of organizations and millions of individuals worldwide.

Mark is a prolific writer with many bestselling books in addition to the *Chicken Soup for the Soul* series. Mark has had a profound influence in the field of human potential through his library of audios, videos, and articles in the areas of big thinking, sales achievement, wealth building, publishing success, and personal and professional development. He is also the founder of the MEGA Seminar Series.

Mark has received numerous awards that honor his entrepreneurial spirit, philanthropic heart, and business acumen. He is a lifetime member of the Horatio Alger Association of Distinguished Americans.

You can reach Mark at www.markvictorhansen.com.

Amy Newmark is the publisher and editor-in-chief of *Chicken Soup for the Soul*, after a 30-year career as a writer, speaker, financial analyst, and business executive in the worlds of finance and telecommunications. Amy is a *magna cum laude* graduate of Harvard College, where she majored in Portuguese, minored in French, and traveled extensively. She and her husband have four grown children.

After a long career writing books on telecommunications, voluminous financial reports, business plans, and corporate press releases, Chicken Soup for the Soul is a breath of fresh air for Amy. She has fallen in love with Chicken Soup for the Soul and its life-changing books, and really enjoys putting these books together for Chicken Soup's wonderful readers. She has co-authored three dozen *Chicken Soup for the Soul* books and has edited another two dozen.

You can reach Amy through the webmaster@chickensoupforthesoul.com.

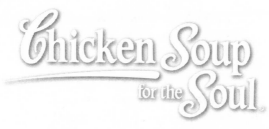

About Richard Simmons

Delivering a serious message with his trademark humor, Simmons, the nation's most revered fitness expert, has helped millions of overweight men and women lose close to 3,000,000 pounds by adopting sensible balanced eating programs and exercise regimes that are energetic, fun and motivating.

Growing up in the French Quarter of New Orleans, where lard was a food group and dessert mandatory, Richard was at 268 pounds when he graduated high school. After trying everything from bizarre diets to laxatives, Simmons took control of his weight problem by adopting a lifestyle of balance, moderate eating and exercise.

Simmons relocated to Los Angeles in 1973. There was no significant fitness movement in this country at the time, and Simmons could not find a health club for people who were not already in shape. His only alternative was to create that safe haven himself. In 1974, after consulting with doctors and nutritionists to ensure the safety of a program tailored to the needs of everyone, he established an innovative place where the overweight of the world were welcomed with open arms. This program met with instant success and continues today at Slimmons in Beverly Hills, where Richard still teaches. While many of his legions of fans are overweight, he also resonates with anyone who has a few pounds to lose and wants to be fit.

Simmons' success as a fitness expert and advocate led to numerous local and national television and radio appearances including a four-year run on *General Hospital*, followed by his own nationally syndicated series, *The Richard Simmons Show*. The show ran for four years and received several Emmy Awards.

Knowing that exercise and weight loss regimes must go hand in hand, Simmons has created a series of products that integrate the two components of a sensible weight loss program. Deal-A-Meal and the FoodMover help people keep track of their food intake through the use of a device to keep track of calories and portions. His *Sweatin' to the Oldies* videos combine lively music with rockin' routines and Simmons' humorous banter and encouragement.

As the author of nine books, including the *New York Times* bestseller, *Never Say Diet*, Richard released his autobiography, *Still Hungry—After All These Years* in 1999. He is also the author of three bestselling cookbooks.

Still fighting the fitness battles with humor and enthusiasm, Simmons vows to never give up. He will continue his crusade until it's time for him to teach classes at the Pearly Gates. You can visit Richard Simmons at richardsimmons.com to read more about him and his programs and products.

Thank You

We owe huge thanks to all of our contributors. We know that you poured your hearts and souls into the thousands of stories and poems that you shared with us, and ultimately with each other. We appreciate your willingness to open up your lives to other Chicken Soup for the Soul readers. And we loved hearing about how you manage your own diet and fitness programs. As we worked on this book, our whole publishing staff found that we were eating better, discussing healthy choices, and exercising more. I personally started eating an apple every day and taking the stairs the three floors from our parking garage to our office.

We could only publish a small percentage of the stories that were submitted, but we read every single one and even the ones that do not appear in the book had an influence on us and on the final manuscript. Thank you so much for sharing your stories on such a personal topic!

Putting together this book was a team effort. I especially thank our editor Kristiana Glavin who read all the stories that were submitted for this book and narrowed down the thousands of submissions to several hundred for me to consider. Our assistant publisher, D'ette Corona, our webmaster and editor, Barbara LoMonaco, and our editor Madeline Clapps worked hard on organizing the manuscript and proofreading it along the way to the printer.

Working with Richard Simmons was a joy and an inspiration. Yes, Richard, I will try to do some straight-leg pushups—at least one!

We owe a very special thanks to our creative director and book producer, Brian Taylor at Pneuma Books, for his brilliant vision for our covers and interiors. Finally, none of this would be possible without the business and creative leadership of our CEO, Bill Rouhana, and our president, Bob Jacobs.

~Amy Newmark, Publisher

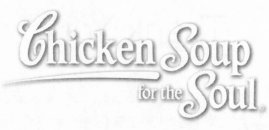

Improving Your Life
Every Day

Real people sharing real stories—for 17 years. Now, Chicken Soup for the Soul has gone beyond the bookstore to become a world leader in life improvement. Through books, movies, DVDs, online resources and other partnerships, we bring hope, courage, inspiration and love to hundreds of millions of people around the world. Chicken Soup for the Soul's writers and readers belong to a one-of-a-kind global community, sharing advice, support, guidance, comfort, and knowledge.

Chicken Soup for the Soul stories have been translated into more than forty languages and can be found in more than one hundred countries. Every day, millions of people experience a Chicken Soup for the Soul story in a book, magazine, newspaper or online. As we share our life experiences through these stories, we offer hope, comfort and inspiration to one another. The stories travel from person to person, and from country to country, helping to improve lives everywhere.

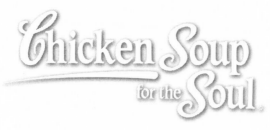

Share with Us

We all have had Chicken Soup for the Soul moments in our lives. If you would like to share your story or poem with millions of people around the world, go to chickensoup.com and click on "Submit Your Story." You may be able to help another reader, and become a published author at the same time. Some of our past contributors have launched writing and speaking careers from the publication of their stories in our books!

Our submission volume has been increasing steadily—the quality and quantity of your submissions has been fabulous. We only accept story submissions via our website. They are no longer accepted via mail or fax.

To contact us regarding other matters, please send us an e-mail through webmaster@chickensoupforthesoul.com, or fax or write us at:

Chicken Soup for the Soul
P.O. Box 700
Cos Cob, CT 06807-0700
Fax: 203-861-7194

One more note from your friends at Chicken Soup for the Soul: Occasionally, we receive an unsolicited book manuscript from one of our readers, and we would like to respectfully inform you that we do not accept unsolicited manuscripts and we must discard the ones that appear.

Chicken Soup for the Soul

www.chickensoup.com